Seven Wheelchairs

Seven | WHEELCHAIRS |

A Life beyond Polio   Gary Presley

UNIVERSITY OF IOWA PRESS, IOWA CITY

University of Iowa Press, Iowa City 52242
Copyright © 2008 by the University of Iowa Press
www.uiowapress.org
Printed in the United States of America

Text design by Omega Clay

The University of Iowa Press is a member of Green Press Initiative and is committed to preserving natural resources.

Printed on acid-free paper

Library of Congress Cataloging-in-Publication Data
Presley, Gary.
    Seven wheelchairs: a life beyond polio / by Gary Presley.
    p.   cm.
    ISBN-13: 978-1-58729-693-2 (clothbound)
    ISBN-10: 1-58729-693-4 (clothbound)
    1. Presley, Gary—Health. 2. Poliomyelitis—Patients—United States—Biography. 3. People with disabilities—United States—Biography. I. Title.
    RC181.U5P74 2008
    362.196'8350092—dc22   2008010014
    [B]

08 09 10 11 12 C 5 4 3 2 1

Title page photo copyright Kenneth C. Zirkel

To Belinda,
friend, lover, life-giver, and soul-mate

Jon,
brother and friend

Verdie B. and Erlyne Pope Presley,
with love and honor

Acknowledgments

This memoir began as an essay, a first-person piece about the days, weeks, months—time that still remains imprecisely measured for me—I spent in an iron lung, that antiquated device at once so fearsome and so necessary, meant to keep alive people with respiratory insufficiency.

I wrote the essay because one of my writer heroes is Richard Selzer. I wrote it in imitation of his essays about his work as a physician.

I was then a member of an online writing critique group, the Internet Writing Workshop. I posted the essay there for other members to critique.

"You need to write a book," was a common response. And so I did, banging out twenty or thirty thousand words during a week at a cabin my wife, Belinda, built near the little town of Shell Knob on the shores of Table Rock Lake in southern Missouri's Ozark Mountains.

Initially, this book was a series of linked essays, all attempting to answer the questions people really want to ask after they discover I've used a wheelchair for nearly fifty years. Many of those short works were critiqued by the IWW's nonfiction group, and to its members I owe sincere appreciation. Their kind words of support and thoughtful suggestions have made this memoir a real thing, a living story, a meaningful history of one life.

As I gained confidence, many people whom I respect suggested the book would work better as a narrative. I turned to Jeannette Cezanne of Customline Wordware, who helped me discover that, yes, there was a sequential narrative story to be found by reframing the essays.

Others supported me in less material but no less helpful ways. I owe significant thanks to Grace Skibicki and Kathleen Purcell, both of whom have read and reread the manuscript in its many forms, always responding with keen and knowledgeable comments. They have been accurate in their criticism and ever-patient with my demands. My friends Grace and Kathleen are accomplished writers and long-time administrators of the Internet Writing Workshop, where they have dedicated innumerable volunteer hours to managing the cooperative that serves so many so well.

Other members of the IWW deserve recognition for consistently challenging me, never letting me decide to skip another rewrite or believe that I am not compelled to tell all the truths I can discover. I will mention Paul Pekin, Peggy Vincent, Sarah Morgan, Diane Diekman, Rich Maffeo, Barbara Mullins, Dawn Goldsmith, Mona Vanek, Ross Eldridge, Karna Converse, Bob Sanchez, Carter Jefferson, and Ruth Douillette among countless others with whom I've interacted personally over the decade I have been a member and administrator of the IWW. I am grateful for every gesture of support and friendship from those named, and from others not listed here.

A rare few of us succeed without support of family. Matthew and Christopher Baldwin, my stepsons, have been patient when writing pulls me away. My brother, Jon, and his wife, Linda, whom I cherish more as a sister than a sister-in-law, along with their daughter Karin and son James, also have cheerfully supported my efforts. My wife's family—her dear mother Joyce DeCamp, her sister Roxane Hill, and her father and his wife, Michael and Nancy Livery—have encouraged me by laughing in the right places after reading some of my comic essays.

But it is my wife, Belinda, who reads what I write with her heart, and, when my words touch that dear place, I know I have found the right words. Any success I have as a writer has been inspired by Belinda.

To find a publisher is a difficult enterprise, one that began for me by mailing query letters, proposals, and sample chapters to agent after agent. It was only after I began querying independent presses and university presses did I discover the fine work accomplished by the University of Iowa Press. I found the editor-in-chief's name through the Internet and shipped a query and two chapters of this memoir to her. I mailed the package on Thursday, and the following Tuesday I received an e-mail from the editor, Holly Carver, asking for the complete manuscript.

It is to Holly Carver, who has been a virtual well of enthusiastic support, that I owe unending gratitude. That my saga is now printed within the covers of a book—that you hold in your hands a story that shows that a life disabled is a life worth living, worth celebrating—is Holly's achievement as much as it is mine. To Holly, to acquisitions editor Joseph Parsons, and managing editor Charlotte Wright, I offer thanks beyond my ability to express in words. I also thank Lisa Raffensperger for her intelligent copy-edits; and any errors that remain are mine.

This book is a memoir, a hard-earned narrative, about a seventeen-year-old boy on the cusp of manhood, sat down to live out the remainder of his life using a wheelchair. Names have been changed, at least a good number of them. I prefer not to embarrass people who cannot speak for themselves. If people read lines that are less than flattering and believe the words were written with animosity and intention to injure, I say that is not so. All that has happened to me—whether I then perceived it for good or ill—gave me the power and insight to write this book and the intent to remember Mark Twain's words: "Kindness is a language which the deaf can hear and the blind can see."

I also beg indulgence from good friends like Father Allan Saunders, Richard and Eileen Henderson, and others who are identified by name.

Of course, the conversations you will read are re-created. They are the words that flowered in my memory as I wrote my story. The incidents and anecdotes—and the memories—are as true as I know how to make them.

I do believe in Truth—that the Infinite One's creation seeks its ordained end—but I believe each of us lives within our separate truths.

I have written this memoir as I have remembered things I perceived and observed, but I realize that how I felt about those people and places and perceptions—or at least, how I interpret them as I write—differs from the stories others might tell.

I am content to chase the mirage of my life in this memoir, only wanting to remind you that sometimes, in the words of Jean-Paul Sartre, "Like all dreamers, I mistook disenchantment for truth."

Seven Wheelchairs

1

I want to remember that final step toward my destiny, that one pace forward to stand under the needle.

I watched the point descend toward my arm, and I turned away. I know I was wearing Levi's. I always wore Levi's. Was I wearing my favorite black cowboy boots, the ones that had prompted the local kids to nickname me Tex? I wasn't nervous. I wasn't fearful. I had taken dozens of inoculations. I had grown past worrying about the minuscule pain, but I remained a bit skittish about the idea of being stuck, and so I never watched the needle penetrate my skin.

Dr. Capetti struck.

I felt the sting. Only a sting then, but it was an unspoken promise of pain I cannot describe, not even now.

I would walk seven days more, only seven days, and then I would be lifted into an iron lung and walk never again.

2

Seven days after taking that final inoculation in the Salk vaccine, I began to burn with poliomyelitis—both types—lumbar and bulbar.

The booster shot was supposed to be a live but attenuated virus, made up of billions of parasites looking for a host, but it gave me the disease because the killed virus inoculations—the first of a series of Salk's miraculous, life-preserving inoculations—hadn't produced antibodies as it was meant to do, and so my body was left defenseless in the face of the nerve-destroying invaders.

There was a time when I cared about that inoculation, about the paralysis it launched into my veins, and I sought someone, something, to blame. Early on, I never failed to confront physicians I encountered. Most denied the possibility that the Salk vaccine had given me polio. Others nodded their heads when I voiced my theory and then moved on to other subjects. Over the decades, doctors would forever be evasive or silent, treating the results rather than the cause, ignoring the imperfection of science, rationalizing what could not be changed or even explained. Doctors are overly busy, after all. Why waste time discussing one insignificant failure among miracles of medicine, a thing that inflicted only a single hurt that can never be healed?

Years later, I learned there were one or two manufacturers that produced flawed vaccines, but the reports say those errors occurred before 1959, the year I lined up for that final shot.

I don't regret, I think, taking the inoculation. I regret most how I responded, how I wasted years not understanding what I had not lost, how I was too unsophisticated to comprehend that we are not so much our ever-changing physical selves but rather our own creation—a being we construct by striking attitude with the hammer of experience.

It matters not how we move through the world. It matters only that we are in the world.

Push me, though, and I will admit I wish I had walked down that line two or three decades later, during the time when an ambitious attorney in litigious society might smell the drug companies' blood in the water. I would rather be rich and crippled than . . .

. . . cynical and unfeeling, a burnt-out case, which I attempted—attempt—to explain away by saying I survived then and I survive now by mating an ignorant combination of existentialism and stoicism, by becoming a peculiar bastardized oddity rolling about the world, forever dependent.

Of course, it is madness to regret what cannot be changed, and I now have learned to keep the madman locked away where he cannot hurt anyone.

3

I am awake. I am alert. But all that was normal has been locked away.

I am in an iron lung. The fever of polio and pneumonia have burnt me down to the ashes of self. I have yet to decide if I will rise up out of the cinders to begin again. I have yet to learn that I am only a remnant of that person I had been shaping into me.

My progress from the confusion of fever down into oblivion, and then up to a different reality, has been seamless. I can draw no line. I can find no border between the real and the unimagined. Somewhere in the circles of light to dark, and then light to dark again, and once more and again, I begin to feel the seductive rhythm of an iron lung. My parents, the doctors, and the nurses explain where I am. Once. Twice. Once more. And then again.

I remember seeing an iron lung in the hallway while I waited in an emergency room, my legs paralyzed. How many days ago? No one says. Is this the same device? No, it can't be. This is a different hospital. I recall an ambulance and the bumpy, shifting, swaying nervousness I felt, stretcher dipping and tilting, as it was lifted, rolled, and carried. An ambulance. Yes, I was being moved—I knew that. From Baptist Hospital to another hospital, one I would learn days later was called Burge Protestant Hospital.

"Careful. Don't let me fall," I said then.

Now I say, "I'm awake. You can let me out, okay? I don't want to be in this thing."

A nurse says, "No. Not right now, hon. You need a little help with your breathing."

I cannot see her, but I believe her. I stop. Focus. Attempt to think.

But I am tired, so tired I can barely move my fingers. Wait. I can move my fingers, a bit, one or two on each hand, but I can't move my arms.

I feel the pressure of the great lung; I feel it release. I do not ask again for them to open the machine and let me try to breathe naturally. I am tired, too tired to fight, tired enough to know I have lost, but not what I have lost. I do what I am told.

I am unable to breathe, the machine reminds me—hum, flap, thump!—sixteen times a minute. They say I can't walk. I remember, yes. That's why I'm here. I couldn't get out of bed that morning . . . when? Days. A week?

Even though I'm too weak now to move my arms, so weak I can only flutter my fingers, I can feel my legs, waiting, impatient to escape the pain that scorches down my spine. I will move one now, yes. I feel the impulse surge to my toes, but nothing happens. I feel dead. Trapped. Mind racing. Body still.

Why?

I could walk. What's wrong? I could run. I could run a mile, sucking in air to drive my legs, running past the pain in my ribcage, running with purpose, running toward a destination, running out of joy.

I am awake, and then tired once more. I am out of kilter with the clock-regulated world. Light reflects through the curtain, and then no light. Lights beyond my head burn continuously, beyond where I rest flat on my back. No matter when I open my eyes, I am greeted by their glow. I drift, awake, asleep, always exhausted, always hurting too badly to drop off into the darkness completely.

"Nurse, can I have something for the pain?"

"Wait till the doctor calls in. We'll get you a hypo."

Machine rhythm infuses the pain in my back, hips, and legs, flowing in, flowing out, fingering the nerves constantly. I feel the great cylinder vibrate imperceptibly, below the level of sound. I begin to listen to the beast, take in its metallic smell, feel it mindlessly working even when I think of other things.

I begin to believe in it, trust it to keep me safe, hiding within its core, humbled and defeated.

The iron lung hums, electric, like a refrigerator or a clothes dryer. The drone is low-pitched, constant. Over that, there is a plaid pattern of other noises—a flap, a sigh, a mechanical flexing, and then another flap as the sequence begins once more. Its mechanics—motor, piston, bellows—palpitate. The soft collar around my neck flutters with the beat, and my chest expands and contracts as the lung carries on its lonely dance.

Iron machine, soft collar, burnt-up body.

Now, flushed by the virus, I see only the great metal circle which surrounds my neck, the cap on the tube more than three feet in diameter, my face—yes, my face, I'm sure, although it is not me, instead a gaunt reflection of my shadow—resting in a mirror hanging above me. I fly through dreams, through sleep, through the odd uncountable waking hours, as part of a huge machine, cumbersome, heavy, and thoroughly unnatural in its appearance.

It is a lung in practice, but a robot lung surrounding a human body rather than a fleshy one inside the body.

Be human . . . muscles surround the chest cavity to expand the ribcage and create a negative pressure. Air flows in, bringing oxygen to burn.

Be human . . . lungs dormant, muscles alienated, left unfired by a short-circuited neurosystem.

Be human, afraid . . . and live on, live inside a pseudo-lung, a steel cylinder perhaps seven feet long by three feet in diameter. Live on, within God's tool, this divine machine, this metal being with a life-sustaining vacuum at its core.

I breathe, or rather the machine forces me to breathe, and so there is no line of demarcation. I breathe now, lung-encased, and I do not remember not breathing. I remember illness, the emergency room, and the hushed, urgent voices of my parents talking with doctors and nurses, but I cannot recall the point when the physicians said I must be placed in the machine.

Did I cry after the decision was made and the end-cap was locked down? Or did they give me sufficient morphine so that I would submit without struggle? That most natural of acts, that involuntary firing of nerve ends and muscles, all that which sets a human being to breathing unconsciously has been swept away. No death is possible by choosing not to breathe—we can hold our breath until we faint, but our bodies will prevail, will not accept the choice of death, will instead suck in air after will has diminished in unconsciousness.

Until polio.

And then all goes awry, and the electrochemical engine is skewed by a minuscule virus.

Never mind. I am safe now, at least so the doctors and nurses tell me. "Relax. Everything's going to be all right."

My body has failed me, but the machine will not allow me to die. The only necessity is that I submit to its functioning.

I have lost the use of my body and control over its function, and I have lost the memory of their theft.

Soon I sleep fewer hours and begin to assess this new world and my place in it. I talk little. I remain weak; even the effort to speak seems to drain me. And I must obey the direction of the machine when I want to speak. It pumps, and it releases, and my speech marches to its cadence. I speak in snatches, in partial sentences, in brief thoughts as it lifts me to exhalation.

"Can someone . . ."

The iron beast cranks, flaps, and sighs.

". . . get me a . . ."

Another cycle.

". . . drink of water?"

I am ultrasensitive to every touch. I even feel the odd little shift in air pressure tickle my skin when a nurse or an aide opens one of the access ports to tend me. The nerves along the top of my thighs burn constantly; with portholes ajar, I sense cooling air but get no relief.

Another day passes. Or two. Perhaps three or four. Or more. Time does not require that I measure it, only that I endure it.

I arrive at the day when I will learn all that once was simple is now complex.

4

I need a bath. There is sweat and dead skin to scrub, but I will cease breathing if the iron lung is opened so that my body may be cleaned thoroughly. The bath begins with a call to the hospital's respiratory therapy department. A technician is sent with a positive pressure machine, complete with mask to be strapped over my face to feed me air.

"He's on his way," says a nurse as she enters my room. "It's going to be that goofball, Ray." She will direct the group of aides gathered near my iron lung waiting for the therapist and his machine.

It is time for a bath and time for a lesson. The bath will cleanse me. The lesson will sketch out the borders between life and death in this inhospitable new country, this devastated land to which I have been exiled.

Ray, the therapist, enters the room, and he grabs control of the situation, overbearingly cheerful. "Bath time, huh? Let's get started."

Ray is dressed head to toe in white—white slacks, a white open-collared shirt, and white shoes. The only color evident is a black leather belt and his dark, crewcut hair. All white, and all business. The group stands beside the iron lung, and Ray moves to the machine's head, quickly strapping a mask to my face and clicking on the portable positive pressure ventilator he has brought with him.

The air that I breathe turns inside out.

I am no longer part of the machine, a fragile blood-circulating core sucking in air to burn. I become the subject of an external device, a flesh balloon to be force-fed air carrying life-sustaining oxygen.

The portable respirator whistles, and a shot of air inflates the mask and squeezes my face. Seven hundred cubic centimeters thrust down my throat at fifteen pounds of overpressure. The pump will sustain life while I am washed, dried, and powdered. Sixteen times a minute.

The aides open the latches that seal the iron lung. In seconds I'm out, my cot pulled from the cylinder. Cool air. Two of the group step to each side of the cot. Warm water. Antiseptic soap. Washcloths. They busy themselves, and Ray wanders out the door.

I'm clean, the front at least, and I'm turned up on my right side so the left half of my back can be washed. The nurses and aides chatter. I have nothing to say, and no way to say it. I am gagged, muffled, with the mask extending from under the chin to over my nose.

The positive pressure machine spews air, clicks valves, spews again. Sixteen times a minute I am reminded that I am no longer whole, no longer a body able to sustain itself and no longer the me who lives within its fleshy organism, its reality.

I cannot bathe. I cannot breathe.

In the lung, I am machine, the brain at its center. I give myself over to its measured beat, and I think, I speak, I sleep. I am secure in the lung, a steel tank, my head poking through its turret to direct all who approach. In the lung, I draw in air to sustain me like every other human being ever born, although as helpless as an armored medieval knight toppled from his horse.

Now, free of my shell, exposed, twisted and turned, being handled briskly, I feel air forced upon me by this new device, banging into my nostrils and mouth and down my throat.

Dog on a leash, fish on a line.

All that I am, or rather all that I have left of me, dangles at the end of a plastic hose. There is a threat implicit in the rigid, overpowering mechanical dominance of this little gadget on rollers, all cool stainless steel and unblinking gauges, standing by my head.

And then suddenly there is nothing.

The nurses and aides rotate me from right side to left side. My head flops and jerks the mask connection off of the feeder tube.

No air.

I fall, as if I slipped from the edge of a cliff, falling into the raw new me, the one who can suck in only a few miserably inadequate cubic centimeters of air by a panicked constriction of his throat muscles.

God! Essential air gone, oxygen deprivation immediate. Such a slender, fragile link to the world, this air, this invisible gas spewing on the floor.

I feel my heart, my eyes. I feel my tongue. There is the pain of my skeleton being flexed as the aides continue to scrub me. But all that cannot be real, for I am locked down, pulled under to where there is no air.

A weight presses in, clamps hard, harder, not on my lungs but upon my whole body. I am seized. A heaviness, as if some great thing squeezes my chest, and from somewhere deep inside me its absolute opposite—the sucking pressure of a vacuum. Weight and vacuum, two forces pushing, pulling, holding me locked breathless between them.

The alarm on the portable respirator emits a solid tone. What has been a soft, intermittent beep marking each blast of air becomes a steady trill, a steamkettle whistle signifying trouble.

The nurse and aides ignore it.

Can't they hear it over their chatter? The noise plays on, a one-note background song to their inattention, to their objectification of my body as a piece of work to be accomplished, to their talk of children and husbands, weather and vacations. I cannot breathe. I panic. I flick my fingers against an unseen arm.

"What's wrong with him?" the aide I touch asks. She looks around the cap of the iron lung machine, but she sees nothing amiss. The mask remains on my face. She does not look at the respirator and see the dangling hose. She does not look into my eyes and see the fear trembling in the pupils.

"You got me," another one replies. "You know how he is. Always complaining about hurting or being uncomfortable."

The first one, my chance for help, looks around the top again. "Don't worry. We know it's not easy for you, but you've got to get used to these baths."

I have no breath to make a noise and reach outside the mask. Instead I emit a low, primitive grunt, a sound elemental, a sound not vocalized but rather drawn from my body as it begins to shut down.

No one notices. I can feel their hands upon me. I can hear the alarm. Surrounded by four people, I am alone, and I cannot breathe. I am aware, but I am powerless.

Thirty seconds? A minute? Ray, the respiratory therapist, skids through the door and immediately notices the machine's hose loose upon the floor.

"What's your hurry?" asks a nurse.

"That's the warning alarm," he says. He reattaches hose to mask.

Air! I suck in air. The room expands. I feel my heart lurch toward normalcy. I gulp. Ray and the women bathing me begin to sort through the confusion.

"We just thought the noise was part of what the machine . . ."

"I was up at the nursing station when I heard it, and I thought one of you would look . . ."

As they mutter excuses and shift responsibility and blame, Ray and the nurse reassemble the iron lung and set it again to its work. Ray reaches to free me of the mask.

"Where the hell . . ." I wait momentarily for the iron machine to draw air enough to give voice to rage.

". . . were you?"

Even my anger is mechanical, ever the slave to the next beat. "And them!"

Another pause.

"I'm trying to tell them I . . ."

Once again, the beat.

". . . can't breathe, and they . . ."

Another pause. The bellows pump, and I can display my anger again.

"Shit! God damn! I could have died."

"You weren't going to die," he replied. "I heard the alarm, and I came running."

But I knew better.

I understood polio had pushed me beyond the edge of my body's ability to sustain itself, that to stay alive I would need to be aware of all that might trip me, defensive against those who cannot see the peril, and ready always to seize control. I had become something more than human and something less.

A bird that cannot fly remains a bird. I will live in the air, but I will never again be able to fly. I cannot draw in air enough to lift me up again, to be Gary. Will there always be a machine and a hose? And will there always be a Ray, me his dependent?

Lord God, I do not want to die. I am afraid. I am paralyzed: the brainstem's perfection of the subconscious, the involuntary acquiescence to thrive by drawing oxygen remains, but its agents, nerves, muscles, are gone now, forever. I am left to go on about the business of living.

My mother visits the next day and I tell her the story. She rubs my forehead and bends down to kiss me. My voice shakes, and then I become angry. "Those stupid bastards could have killed me."

"Don't swear," she replies. "You're all right now. These people are trained for emergencies."

I know otherwise, but I cannot yet voice what I learned: I will never live another day without thinking about being able to breathe.

5

The war for my body began with a headache, one that came from the core, from a knife-point deep in the triangle where the spine meets brain and brain meets eyes.

"I'm taking the bus home," I said to the coach. "I'm sick." I dropped the basketball and walked toward the exit to the gym. Basketball practice was over for me.

The headache was notice that my world had turned upside down, that a strange journey was underway, but it really didn't begin there. Nor had it begun the instant the needle carrying that last in the series of polio vaccines penetrated my skin a week before.

Family history played a part, with the journey beginning in the 1930s, perhaps in a darkened theater in a little town outside of Los Angeles. My grandfather was an oil field roustabout, caught up by the Great Depression like every other working man. Pap, as I called him, worked only two or three days a week for Atlantic-Richfield and added a little extra money to the family income by doing maintenance for a Nisei landlord. My mother's family, the Popes, didn't prosper and didn't starve, and my grandmother always found a few pennies so that my mother and her sister and little brother could spend Saturday afternoon at the movies and get ice cream on the way home.

There, in the cool dark of a theater crammed with children waiting impatiently for the double feature, my mother saw the newsreels—war in China, FDR in Washington, and rows of shiny iron lungs cradling children burning with infantile paralysis. Nurses in white. A doctor in the background. A somber voice announcing news of another polio epidemic.

"They'd close the swimming pools when I was a girl," my mother said. "Mama wouldn't let us play with our friends."

Polio, a disease of the central nervous system, was common then, long before Jonas Salk went into his laboratory and came out with a vaccine. Every adult feared it because it seemed to single out children. There seemed to be an epidemic every summer. "Don't get overtired through work, play, exercise, or travel," warned the National Foundation for Infantile Paralysis. "Don't get chilled. Don't use another person's towels, dishes, or tableware. Don't take your children to places where there is polio."

There was no preventive and no cure. Parents knew only that polio could strike their children, leave them unable to move their arms or legs.

Or breathe.

My mother had believed the warnings as a girl, but my mother also grew up with a faith that however hard things became, life would be better tomorrow. She had lived through World War II and welcomed her husband home safe. She had seen penicillin save lives and blood transfusions become routine. She had submitted herself to vaccinations for exotic diseases so that she could travel overseas as the wife of an army officer, and she had come home healthy. And so, in 1956, when the Salk vaccine became available to the general public, my mother took her two sons and joined the long line of her fellow optimists on a windy street in Spokane, Washington.

I was fourteen, and I believed too. All my life, moving from army fort to army fort around the world, I had been inoculated for diseases I could neither spell nor pronounce nor identify. And I had seen the rows of iron lungs in the newsreels and in *Life* magazine and the *Saturday Evening Post*. I didn't fear polio, but I didn't want it.

But I got it. Got it when hundreds of other youngsters, my brother included, didn't. Got it because I had faith in the rightness of things, got it because some quirk in my metabolism misfired, got it because we did all the right things.

6

"My head hurts so bad I can barely see," I said to my father. I had taken aspirin when I arrived home after skipping basketball practice. I had swallowed the pills, complained to my mother as she began dinner, and then joined my father in the barn. Farm animals don't care if you're sick.

Dad was preparing to milk the small dairy herd he'd purchased to support our Missouri farm. My job was to feed the calves, and I was mixing supplement for them. He turned toward me but said nothing for a moment. My father believed in "I can" not "I'll try." But he must have seen something in my appearance that convinced him I wasn't offering an empty excuse to get out of the evening chores.

"Well, go on then," he said. "Go on back to the house and take some more aspirin."

And so I began my final journey on foot. I can see the whitewashed wooden fence surrounding the corral, the woven wire enclosing the garden, the slope of the path angling slightly uphill toward the back door of our house. It was a hundred yards, perhaps, from the milking parlor in the bow-top Dutch barn and across the muddy feedlot, dodging manure piles, then through the fall remnants of my mother's garden, and onto the porch of our rock house half a mile from Spring Creek, three miles north of where the creek joined the James River, and then into the waters of the Arkansas River basin, and finally sweeping into the great Mississippi and out to sea.

Sea legs.

There's no better way to describe the feeling, the way the earth touched me through my feet, as I made that last walk. Every footfall dropped with a dizzy awkwardness, the same mushy unsureness at the ankle and knee of a sailor long at sea taking his first steps on land. I had been to sea. I knew.

But I did not know what would await my return.

"What's wrong, Gary?" my mother asked. "Are you that sick?"

"I really don't feel good, Mom. Dad said I better come take more aspirin."

I did and found my way to my bed, one step, two, through the kitchen and hallway and into the room I shared with my brother, Jon. I must have removed my boots and jeans, but . . .

I felt someone shaking me. "Time to get up. Let's get down to the barn," my father said.

Morning? Yes. My head hurt still, but I swung my legs over the side of the bed and pushed myself up.

And fell on my face.

I yelled, and my father came running to stand over me. "My legs don't work," I said.

"What's happening?" My mother had entered the room, tying her robe around her.

"I don't know," said Dad. "He says he can't stand. Help me get him back on the bed."

Strange, I thought. Stranger still now, I remember, for I wasn't panicked. I was confused. Why wouldn't my legs work? Everything else seemed okay. I could see. I could hear. When things went wrong physically, I expected pain. In the past I had broken my nose. Painful. I had dislocated my thumbs. Cuts. Bruises. Not quite as painful. But pain was strangely absent now. Sitting in bed, I tried to raise one leg and then the other. I looked down to see myself bare-chested, wearing shorts. My legs looked perfectly normal, right down to the bitter purple L-shaped scar across my left knee. Baseball injury. That hurt.

As I slumped on the bed, I heard indistinct voices from the kitchen. The volume increased as my father called a neighbor from the telephone in the central hallway, but I still couldn't understand the words.

"Get dressed," my father said, leaning into the room. I didn't ask how. I found the shirt I had worn to school the day before draped across a bedside chair. And then my mother slipped in to help me slide my blue jeans over my legs and slip on my shoes.

A dream.

A reality.

My father on one side. Wade Jackson, the neighbor, on the other. My arms across their shoulders. I see my feet. They drag. One flops forward. We are moving from my room, across the kitchen, and down off the enclosed porch. Missy, the cattle dog, watches Wade warily, confused by the three of us bound together.

"Watch your head," Wade says. We have reached our car.

I'm in the back seat, and we are off to the hospital. The Baptist Hospital in Springfield, Missouri. We know the city, but we know no doctors. Wade has said the Baptist Hospital is the best.

"Ask for Durward Hall," Wade had told my father.

But Dr. Hall does not come to the emergency room. Are we in the hospital basement, this place that bustles? I remember a dim, narrow corridor, a room, and my father prowling. My mother sits opposite the cot where I lay. She wears her coat still, and she seems drawn in upon herself. She is a tall woman with a strong nose and chin, and it is her habit to stand straight and move purposefully. Where is Jon? One of the orderlies mistakes my mother for the sister I do not have. I smile. This is my mother, not a girl. It is October 1959. She is thirty-nine years and three months old. Her life is changing more than she can imagine.

One person after another enters and leaves. I wonder again where Jon is. He's only eight. He needs someone to watch him, help him get to school. I wait. Nothing is done, but it doesn't matter. I feel better, headache diminished, but I still cannot move my legs. I am impatient, but I ask no questions. What is there to ask? My legs do not work, and that seems a mystery beyond explanation. I am seventeen years and five months old, and I have only briefly been acquainted with a paralyzed person, never considered paralysis as a human condition.

I drift, and then I hear, "You'll have to hold him very steady." My father grabs my shoulder and my knees, grips hard, and pulls me on to my side. A man I cannot see sends a needle into my spine to seek a sample of that which has brought me here. The doctor's name, I will learn later, is Thomas Cochran, and he is an internist and a partner in a clinic with Dr. Hall, who is a surgeon.

I do not remember Dr. Cochran entering the room, but he has taken control. My eyes seek my father's face, but he is intent upon the syringe, upon the fluid being drawn from his firstborn. I think now he was repeating to himself, "Not meningitis. Anything but meningitis." Meningitis killed my father's next older brother—Gordon Gilliam Presley, dead at age three.

"Buddy, what are we going to do?" my mother asks after the doctor and his attendants leave. My father says nothing. He simply reaches out to touch her.

Then I see it. Two orderlies in white are moving it down the hall past the room where we wait. A long tube, seven or eight feet perhaps, round, on square legs resting on casters, a pale unhealthy yellow, putrid yellow, in color. One man pulls. The other pushes. I see it, and then it is gone. An iron lung.

"They're not getting me in that thing!" I say. My father insists it is for someone else.

Confusion, voices. Hours uncounted, only endured. An ambulance. I am to be transferred to another hospital by ambulance. Who will pay, I think. Money is important, and we are people who get ourselves to a doctor crawling, refusing to give in, even if we are broken or bleeding. From the ambulance—stops, turns, backing—I am taken into another large brick building and lifted into a bed. I have forgotten about the iron lung. I have left it behind. I sleep, dreamless or dreams unremembered. I awake. My mother is still there, and my father. I am too disoriented to imagine their confusion, their worry, their pain.

Do I ask, "Who's doing the milking?" Perhaps. My father is there, and the cows must be milked twice a day or their udders might rupture. Like my bladder. I cannot urinate. An orderly comes with a catheter.

And then I cannot breathe, and the order comes for me to enter the iron lung.

"No! No! I'm not going in there!" Did I say that aloud? How could I, if I could not breathe? But I am not going into the lung. No, no.

My mind works—does it really, or do I only imagine being lifted?—and so do my hands, but there are several people surrounding me, and they are stronger, and my father is there, and I never disobey my father, at least in his presence. Never. I am being lifted, and I see the iron lung yawning in anticipation, its end-cap opened and the white-sheeted cot comprising its innards pulled out, like a knife from a sheath, and then I am upon it, upon the cot. And I am lifted again, and my head is pushed up through an opening in the end-cap, and then the great device is reassembled and locked together.

I enter my home for the next three months.

I am thrust into the cocoon from which I will metamorphose into he who will never walk again.

I become part of the machine, and I turn myself over to it.

7

By the time the polio flamed out and I'd dug myself out of a pneumonia pit, I began to comprehend that my world had shrunk drastically. I spent every day, all day, on my back in the iron lung—my world was encased within a metal tube in a room I never left in a hospital I never knew existed. No one entered my world without purpose. Orderlies, aides, and nurses sustained me, accomplished chores like tending to food and water, urine and feces. My parents encouraged me.

The doctors were the strangest of all; distant and seemingly useless, they were observers, directors of actions without consequence. Dr. Cochran, or those substituting for him, examined me, said a few harmless words, offered a prescription for painkillers, and left. I know now each felt impotent. What use is medical school in the face of irreversible paralysis? I wanted promises, conviction that I would rise and walk again. I wanted the physicians who relied less on science and experience and believed more in magic, in redemption, in miracles. Instead they lingered a few minutes and then discovered it was time to see the next patient.

The doctors left me to explore a new world, one narrowed to a small window and slice of hallway framed by the door, and a small black-and-white television reflecting the world I had left behind.

Nearly all of it—all of my world—resided within the framework of my iron lung's single passenger accessory—a mirror, six by twelve inches maybe, mounted on a rack perhaps twelve inches above my face. These measurements are approximate. I didn't have a ruler.

When I wanted the mirror tilted this way or that, I asked one of the staff or flagged someone walking along the hall. I had always been the sort of guy to do something myself rather than ask for help. I had been shy and diffident in spite of my cosmopolitan upbringing, and now I found myself self-conscious about being so freakishly confined. It took days or weeks before I'd yell for assistance from anyone not dressed in medical whites. Finally, boredom became a disease of its own, and I began to yell at the first passerby whenever I required help. It was always easy enough to know who'd step into the room to tilt the mirror or change the channel or adjust the volume. They were the ones who would walk past the room, see the iron lung, and not rapidly avert their eyes as if they'd just caught a glimpse of their mother naked.

Watching television in a mirror isn't any better than watching it straight on, but it does teach you one thing: how to read when the letters of words and sentences are reversed. The best instructors for that skill were daytime game shows. I liked noitartnecnoC and drowssaP best. My favorites—westerns, sports, and detective shows—didn't require much reading, other than saloon doors and scoreboards. But too much of any one thing is boring, especially since this was pre-cable and the city of Springfield, Missouri, astraddle Route 66 and with a population of 100,000, had only two channels, NBC and CBS.

After my senses returned, I began to read for a good part of the day. One of the staff asked me if I liked to read and then described how the iron lung's mirror could be replaced with a book rack. A book slipped into the rack, and a set of spring-loaded clamps held it open. Two pages read, and one more thing to ask. I would yell for a passerby or a staffer to turn the page and secure it under the clamp. Two more pages, another wait. I made my way through several Dos Passos and Faulkner novels, but I can't tell you which. I have forgotten much of Dos Passos, but I have read Faulkner several times since. I've met some of his Snopeses in my life, and I once became one.

It was there in that hospital, Burge Prostestant in Springfield, Missouri, in its isolation ward where the polio patients were housed, and it was early in my journey, when I was hurt, angry, and full of meaningless, useless self-remorse.

I began to spit on the floor.

I became a Snopes, defiant, self-absorbed, and righteous. I spit out all the anger for others to see.

I spat on the floor for days, perhaps a week or more. I only know I smoldered with a rage that seemed to choke me, and I decided to spit on the floor, and I continued until I decided to stop. I think my life as a Snopes lasted long enough that people began to hate me.

I spat on the floor because I couldn't reach my mouth to wipe away phlegm and mucus with a handkerchief. I was completely paralyzed from my neck down to my toes. But I could still spit.

Not that polio causes an undeniable urge to spit. I spat because I also had had pneumonia. You don't necessarily get pneumonia as a bonus with polio, like some sort of bizarre two-for-one disease sale. You get pneumonia by being too stubborn, or too weak, and by avoiding the exercises and therapies that might prevent your lungs from filling with rancid puddles of infection.

Fate and the failure of the Salk vaccine gave me polio. Ignorance and my unwillingness to endure pain gave me pneumonia.

The blaze of the fever, the inability to move so as to relieve cramps and aches, and the fear—mostly the fear—make polio hurt, and hurt badly. Polio is fire. On the inside. A nasty little virus burning through the central nervous system. Polio is stomach-churning pain, fever aching in the bones and gnawing its way out. It's confusion, and hallucinations, and panic, and anger. The fever burns and the polio paralyzes, and so the simplest, albeit painful, way to avoid pneumonia, the bacterial type that brews in puddles of moisture in the lungs, is to exercise the person fighting polio. Open the iron lung's portholes. Roll the carcass side to side. Roughly slap its back to loosen the fluid turning into gel. Move the polio-paralyzed body regularly, several times a day. Tolerate the inevitable complaints.

"Grit your teeth and stop whining," the therapists told me, "we need to turn you every hour."

Move, and you're a tougher target, not allowing fluid in your lungs to become stagnant water for pneumonia's mosquitoes. The staff came to me those first days, those nurses and orderlies, in the morning, at noon, in the afternoon, and in the evening, and they tried to move me. They explained the necessity of movement, the perils of immobility.

I believed I had learned that lesson already.

The doctor was told I refused to cooperate. "You're never going to get well if you don't change your attitude," he said.

I said, "Stick your ass in this can and then talk to me about attitude."

But not to his face. Instead I continued to cry and complain. The nurses said it had to be done, and they came the next day, and the next. I whined and whimpered. They yelled and demanded compliance, hard words translating into rougher handling. I moaned that it hurt too much.

And I won.

The visits dwindled. First to morning, noon, and night, but I continued to snivel. Soon, it was one visit a day. Or every other day. And as a week passed without me suffering ill effects, they stopped coming by to roll me this way or that, to tilt the iron lung up or down, or to turn me and pound on my back to loosen congestion.

I was paralyzed by polio, and they were paralyzed by their frustration with my self-pity and stubbornness.

I could clench my fists and turn my head, but I could move nothing else, and yet something in my sniveling numbed their good sense. They could not, would not, and finally did not move me. I was paralyzed, and they could walk, but I won. I was weak, and even the smallest of the nurses was strong enough to dominate me, but they walked away and left me alone. I beat them all with my attitude.

I think I have forgiven them. I have never forgiven myself.

Pneumonia arrived in the form of apathy, then fever, and finally delusions. I believed I was locked in a washing machine on my grandparents' farm. I apologized, but no one would set me free. My father told me my grandmother still loved me, and I said, "But she saw me in the machine. Why wouldn't she let me out?"

My room was on the second floor, and I could see the southern horizon, and I remember it as night, for the sky was black but also ablaze with the reflection of the city's lights. I suppose I was at the edge of my own darkness, in a strange place weirdly lit by pneumonia's ravaging fever. The orderlies began clearing the room, pushing the cabinets and chairs into the bright hallway.

A white-clad doctor stepped through the door, surgical cap and gown tied, mask already across mouth and nose.

"Breathe this," he said. He clamped an inhaler over my mouth and nose, and the iron lung began to pump an antiseptic-tasting mist. A numbness crept over my lips and tongue and down my throat.

Anesthetic to numb the mouth and throat, the mind already pneumonia-numbed and too confused to understand the place I would visit that night.

The procedure is called a rigid bronchoscopy. It is accomplished by titling back the patient's head and inserting a hollow tube down the trachea and into each bronchial tube, first one and then the other. In my case, the procedure was undertaken to clear thick mucus blocking my airway. Streptococcus? Staphylococcus? It does not matter; it only means that I had bacterial pneumonia resulting from my refusal of treatment, payback for my cowardly obstruction of every attempt at the necessary painful movements designed to keep my lungs clear of fluid.

I was drowning in my body's excretions, and no one told me how the physicians had decided to rescue me.

Two more doctors and a nurse, gowned and masked, unidentified and unidentifiable, entered. They carried on in the doctor-way—that is, as they pleased, intent on striking the sick nail with their medical hammer. They deflected my mumbled, thick-lipped questions with murmurs and removed the rack that provided a pillow for head and neck support. I hadn't sufficient strength to hold my head level, and so one of them caught it as it snapped down toward the floor. And then he let it flex back further. Then more. Further yet, beyond any point resembling normal. Dear God, it hurt; my head felt as if it would break away and fall to the floor.

I am Doctor. You are Disease.

"Wha . . . ?" I tried to ask.

The white-gowned mob continued without explanation or hesitation. My lungs were to be drained, and the doctors had decided it was to be accomplished with a topical anesthetic rather than a general one. With me somewhat alert, fighting, I could do my part to help by gagging and coughing. Or perhaps they were afraid a general anesthetic would kill me.

It does not matter now. Nor did it matter then.

Tube in.

Impaled.

Sword-swallower.

Tube out.

My head no longer speared through my neck to my gut.

Free to erupt!

First parts of two teeth, shattered when the tube was wrenched from one bronchial tube to the other, and then great yellow-green gelatinous globs of mucus. Finally, breath, precious air, and a spasm of curses.

"You bastards!"

"That's good," said the nearest doctor. "Cough! Get that stuff out."

"You had no right! Son of a bitch! You didn't even ask!"

"Cough harder. Harder! You need to get it all up."

"You broke my goddamn teeth!"

Minutes passed as I coughed and retched, and they stood and watched. Finally, a student nurse entered to clean up the growing mess, and the lung-spearing crew gathered up their instruments and began to filter out the door. I watched as the tall one turned left and moved toward the lounge where my parents waited.

I sobbed more, coughed, retched, and cursed without ceasing. The nurse began to clean my face. She talked quietly, a reassuring murmur, but I had been skewered like a piece of dead meat, and I wanted only to retreat into the pain of my violation.

I coughed all night, the pneumonia beast punctured and dying and seeking release. That which would have killed me after the polio had botched its deadly mission began to bubble up from my chest and soak my pillow.

Throughout the night, a nurse or orderly would answer my call and change the linen, but the morning shift—the busy shift that encompassed breakfasts, baths, and doctor rounds—was less accommodating.

"Hey, my pillow's wet," I said to a nurse scurrying past my door.

"Stop spitting on yourself then. Cough it up and swallow it. It won't hurt you." She hurried on to something or someone more urgent.

"No, I don't . . ." but she had sailed out of my vision.

I would not swallow the refuse. It was poison. It was liquid death. It had choked my lungs. I dared not swallow it where it might pollute my guts. And so once the pillow was soaked, I began spitting on the floor. It was an old hospital, and the floors were tile, the same vile green color as the spit I used to christen them, the same hue as the self-pity still bubbling in my psyche.

Why? I know I spat defiance. I hawked up anger and frustration and spat them onto the floor. *Let them see me suffer.* I spat because I was naked and helpless in a metal tube seven feet long and three feet in diameter, my head exposed like some evil, recalcitrant pilgrim in wooden stocks.

I spat because I could, and no one could stop me.

The days passed, the poison boiled up slowly, the pillow would become soaked and, when the wetness touched my cheek, I would begin spitting on the floor. I could not be dissuaded or bribed or shamed. I stopped only when my mother or father visited, and they reached to wipe the venom from my lips.

No one then worried about HIV or AIDS or Hepatitis C. No one wore a mask or latex gloves. A housekeeper would enter the room, toss a towel on the mess and wipe it up, silent, no word of disapproval. I did not apologize. What's spit compared to vomit, feces, or blood? Why not a towel, a quick swipe, and a quicker departure? Who wants to reason with an emaciated head poking from the end of a seven-foot-long tube on wheels?

Occasionally a nurse would stoop to wipe up the evidence of my insolence. Nurses are never silent.

"Why do you insist on doing this?" said a short, slender one with dark hair. "It's nasty." Her winged starched cap vibrated with disapproval because others were forced to kneel down in homage to my pain and anger.

I did not answer. Nor did I stop spitting on the floor, not that day anyway, not in the face of disapproval.

And then one day I did.

8

The Dodgers and the White Sox played the World Series, the stack of books grew significantly, the television shows bored into routine noise, and Thanksgiving and Christmas passed, both with something to celebrate had I known how or why. But I was still caught up in the drama of being a victim. Days, weeks, of exercises came and went, mostly range of motion lifts and tugs meant to free my stiff joints enough that I might one day fit into a wheelchair.

The physical therapist arrived and pulled my cot from the can. I was to breathe on my own while he attempted to restructure my body. He would first lift my leg by the ankle and knee and attempt to fold it up to touch my chest. One leg. The other. Then up to my arms, his grip at wrist and elbow pulling my arm up far above my head. One arm. The other.

"You'll soon be free of this thing," he said. Free for the first time in weeks. Free to take the next step—from the iron lung and up to sit in a wheelchair for hours, perhaps a whole day, sustained by a respiratory chest shell while upright and by the shell and a rocking bed at night.

I was afraid, but I was ready. I wanted to turn my own pages. And scratch my nose when it itched.

It is the rocking bed I remember most from those midwinter days when the hospital staff began to reassemble my life. Think of a seesaw in a children's playground. Substitute a mattress atop a metal frame for the board, add an electrical motor to accomplish the necessary seesawing at a regular pace, and you have constructed that miraculous contraption. The pace mimics human respiration rates, dipping head down, and then feet down, perhaps fifteen to eighteen times a minute. The idea is that your stomach, liver, and assorted other internal organs bang against the wall of your diaphragm and compress your lungs as the head of the bed dips. That forces air out, and then, when your feet dip, your compressed lungs re-inflate as a vacuum sucking in air.

Two feet up, maybe, and then two feet down. All day, if necessary, and all night, to sustain sleep. Awkward and disconcerting at first— too much blood to the brain and then not enough—but, for me, the rhythm would eventually become soothing, the movement applying gentle pressure to ease the pain of burned-out and abandoned knees and hips and ankles.

The chest shell necessary for my first journey outside the iron lung in more than two months was in fact a miniature half-iron-lung, one to be clamped over my chest, a tiny vacuum chamber that resembled nothing so much as a sea turtle shell. Out of the iron lung, but again to be sustained by the magic of vacuum. The rigid little shell would be strapped securely across my chest, and an electric motor would power a trashcan-size air pump. Vacuum, release. Sixteen times a minute. Yank me into the shell, a gasp of air in response.

All this was necessary because I had greatly diminished respiratory capacity, less than a fourth of normal. On top of that, I was debilitated. The two together—the rocking bed and the chest shell—would assure that my system would continue to function.

An orderly pulled my cot from the iron long, and a respiratory therapist clamped on the chest shell. My weight was down from 165 pounds to perhaps 115, but I was six feet long and could hold neither arms nor legs upright, and they called for help to lift me up from the cot and down into a reclined wheelchair so that I could be moved to the room with the rocking bed.

I became lost in a whirl of dizziness, with my head flopping about on my weakened neck. Arms! Legs! Shriveled! Pale and rough with dead skin—not mine, surely, but look, focus, on how I see—there seem to be—arms and legs radiating down from what I had come to see in my mirror as myself entire: my head and only my head.

Wheelchair, chest shell, and rocking bed—a new world, an old world, all that was me turned near vertical once again, all the looking up becoming looking out, head to balance and sway, legs and arms to flop, spinning away from that which was into that which will be, perhaps, maybe, if only I could see, could hold in the contents of my stomach, could hold my new world still for a moment.

I panicked. I clinched my jaw, felt the tendons and ligaments in my neck tighten and throb as the therapist attached the chest shell. It began to click away, sucking and blowing, but I couldn't catch my breath. The beat was off, and the sensation rough and staccato. I could not cope with the dizziness and the idea that I could exist outside my lung, my home, the engine that had kept me alive for three months. The nurses and orderlies fussed about, muttering reassurances, watching my eyes, asking questions, and forcing me to answer. Gradually my confusion lessened. I wiggled my hand and fingers and watched them move, scaly, crusty, white, rather than my regular darker skin tone.

Then I was rolled into a different room, there to be lifted onto the rocking bed; I was a new being but one still to be acted upon, still dependent, still wary of all that might go awry. Again, panic as I was lifted and tossed onto the rocking bed and the therapist bent to flip the switch that set it into motion.

It darted downward in its first fearsome movement, and my fingers dug into its sheeted mattress as if I had muscle enough to keep from sliding headfirst. The therapist stood alongside as it continued up, down, watching as I crept toward acceptance of the slow, relentless transfer of weight, belly organs squeezing against lungs. Exhale. The bed rose head-up, all that was inside me slid downward, and an artificial vacuum re-inflated my lungs. Soon, after I became comfortable with my surroundings, a physical therapist would take advantage of the nearly unrestricted space for my daily exercise of arms and legs. I submitted, reluctantly at first as always, vocalizing my pain in grunts and murmurs. But then I remembered it would help build strength and endurance—and I liked being free of the lung—so I tried to swallow my complaints. I wanted more time in the wheelchair. I wanted to ride the chair to the physical therapy room and around the ward.

I may not have been free of dependence, but I was freed of the container.

9

"Cool," said Keith. "You're out!"

Keith had sandy hair, with a lock perpetually falling over his right eye. And he smiled and laughed and nearly always seemed in a good mood. He had been closest to me in the hospital—in proximity, anyway—housed in the room adjoining mine. If he had been in an iron lung—I never asked, only assumed—he had progressed to a rocking bed before I became aware of my new place in the world.

Sometimes during the weeks I still required the iron lung, in the quiet after evening visiting hours, an orderly would pull my great yellow beast into the hallway so that I could see into Keith's room. We would talk, him dipping and rising on his rocking bed, me pattering to the rhythm of the lung. He was delighted when I followed him out of the iron lung.

Keith was a tall kid. "I'll be six foot six when they get me off this bed," he said. He had been a star for his high school basketball team. But, like me, he had undergone the polio-weight-loss diet. Keith was significantly underweight, not quite a skeleton, but mostly frame, skin, and constant smile. As with all of us, the disease had zapped both muscle tone and muscle mass.

Now on my rocking bed in the room with Keith, my eyes shifted, bounced, ricocheted from sight to sight, from things new to things familiar, taking in faces and people from a wholly different perspective. After three months stilled, three months horizontal, I began to adjust to motion once more. Free of the iron lung, I was no longer restricted to two views of the world: vertical, left and right, direct to walls and ceilings; or horizontal, but in reverse, contrary to logic.

Instead I moved, up and down with the bed, new perspectives constantly. My delight with all the new images soon overwhelmed any feelings of physical discomfort.

When my graduation from the lung had been announced, I had asked only a few questions. Three months locked within the cylindrical cell had convinced me I was captured. My world would change when others, not me, decided it would change. My choice was to accept or not to accept, but what would be done would be done in spite of that choice.

As I became comfortable with the move to the rocking bed, I also began to understand I had been granted only a pardon from complete confinement to the freedom of a shackle. Nevertheless I felt free. I cannot remember my first night outside the iron lung, but I must have been apprehensive—surrounded by open space, no safety within an armored cylinder, no reflection of my face hovering protectively over me. Then, as today, my fears fed off my ability to breathe. Each time I was taken from the lung for therapy or other reasons, perhaps because of the incident during one of my first baths, I felt a strange claustrophobia, as if I were trapped inside a translucent box. But, within the rhythms of the moving bed and the flexing chest shell, I escaped from the terror of breathlessness. I could not *not* breathe. And Keith was there, a soul to provide an immediate answer if I called out.

Or I may have drifted into sleep because of some subconscious memory of a cradle. It was a place to dread, a rocking bed, but all the same a sanctuary of gentle, comforting, rhythmic movement. I can remember the dip of the bed, head dropping toward the floor, the rush of all that was loose inside me past the point of balance and running rapidly toward my skull. And then the return, my head rocketing upward, and the unfamiliar pressure of weight on my feet locked against a foot-board.

Standing? *Am I standing in my dreams? Will I run?* No, not standing, but a hint of the narrow, focused pressure experienced by every creature that walks the earth—the core of the planet pulling at my feet.

And so I must have given myself over to this different cradle, surrendering to the power of the tireless electric motor, and I slept.

Keith was to leave the hospital long before me. I remember grinning at his image as we said our goodbyes. Paralyzed from only the waist up, he had began to take a few tentative steps shortly after I moved into the room. A therapist and an orderly would stand on either side, and Keith's head would wobble forward. A step. Another. Keith soon found himself taking steps up and down the hallway. I watched as he improved each day, mimicking him by wiggling my left foot—polio's odd little miscue in its attempt to make a new Gary.

The day the doctor set for Keith's release his mother or one of the orderlies had dressed him in his bright green high school letter jacket. Someone had tucked his useless hands into the pockets to keep them from flopping as he walked. His blue jeans were too big then, and his belt was cinched to the last buckle hole.

"I'll be back to visit," he said. He gulped for another breath of air, a conscious effort on his part. "Sometime at least before they kick you out of here." He gulped again, and then again, to fill his lungs with his next breath. The nerves controlling Keith's diaphragm muscles had been damaged or destroyed, and he'd mastered frog-breathing, the art of using throat muscles to force air down the windpipe, to keep his lungs operating. I think every breath he took required a decision or the work of the rocking bed. Every breath was precious, hard-won, and to be used with deliberate calculation.

Keith had been a good temporary friend, the sort I had been familiar with during my life as an army brat, but I didn't expect him to come back for a visit. I had heard "See you soon" from more than one visitor, but only a rare few made good on the casual words. Acquaintances from the little school I had attended for four months after we had moved from El Paso to the farm came once, it seemed, and never returned.

I accepted that as nothing unusual. I had no lifelong friends. This isolation was different, of course, and it took me a while to understand I had embarked on a journey no one wanted to share.

All I know is that I never saw Keith again. Someone told me later he'd died in a hospital emergency room after vomiting blood from a bleeding ulcer. Rumor or truth, I know now the great air-breathing engine that is the human body can be driven only so far before it revolts. Maybe he choked. No diaphragm muscle, no coughing. Aspiration. Death.

Polio can kill you when it strikes. Or later.

. . . .

I had arrived on the last wave of a mini-epidemic marching across southwest Missouri and northern Arkansas. For some reason, those of us stuck in the can—the iron lung—were kept in rooms alone. Maybe it was for morale, to keep from discouraging the other polio patients. If so, that didn't make sense. Once the infection and its fever had run their course, you were about as banged up as you were ever going to be. If a patient had already been through the polio grinder, it wasn't going to give anyone a fit of nerves to see an iron lung in action. And I know it wasn't for public relations, as if the medical staff's egos required the uncomfortable to remain invisible. After all, my room's door was open, and anyone could look in and see me.

But alone in the room after Keith's discharge, I began to notice the difference in responses of people walking down the hallway. I had found it an interesting game while I was in the iron lung to watch passersby and attempt to predict the change in expressions as people caught sight of my head poking from the great yellow cylinder. I was never able to match reaction to appearance. Sometimes a well-dressed, sophisticated-appearing person would say hello or smile; sometimes a guy in overalls might acknowledge me.

Nevertheless, even though I did not want the door to my room closed while I recuperated in the lung, I had always felt as if I were an invisible exhibit, a medical museum piece, a "Damn, poor bastard" to most people, even after I forced acknowledgment or interaction.

Although Keith seemed to like to talk with me, I know I had a reputation among the nurses and aides as a whiner, a difficult and stubborn patient, and so the staff didn't rush to move someone else into the room. I know I felt better, freer; perhaps I complained less. I began to work to expand my world, asking the orderlies, attendants, and nurses about their lives, telling jokes, discussing television shows. I noticed a few people, mostly children, in hospital robes walking the halls. That gave me the idea that maybe I too was free to roam the ward. The only problem was that I was too weak to propel my wheelchair, let alone drag the pump for the chest shell along as a trailer.

I asked one of the orderlies if he'd push me around the ward for a few minutes. He agreed and rolled me to the nurses' station down the hall. That was the first of many trips. Maybe it was because of my improved attitude or maybe it was because the staff said, "Let's get rid of him for a few minutes," but I soon found it easy to convince someone to whisk me out to visit the other long-term residents of the ward.

I had escaped my cocoon, and I became, not a social butterfly, but instead a raggedy moth tethered to a portable respiratory machine as if it were a light.

I visited everyone except Jimmie, the last remaining polio patient in an iron lung cocoon. I was told Jimmie had been hospitalized— cooked by polio and canned by total respiratory dependence—for eleven years. He had the room closest to the nurses' station, and he was popular with the staff. I could see from the hallway that his room was decorated almost like a small studio apartment, appearing not at all like the standard hospital room. He had a large television, a radio, a bookshelf, prints and photographs on the wall, and a comfortable chair for visitors.

I feared him because I did not want to be him, at least any longer. From a place so deep within me that it had no voice, deeper even than my comprehension of my paralysis at the time, I knew that I could have been another Jimmie. I wanted to believe I had escaped the lung forever. Besides, I had nothing to say that would help him. Or me.

Down the hall from Jimmie, there was a small ward meant to accommodate four patients. In it there were three others ahead of me in recovery. All three fought polio and had escaped the battle with only their legs paralyzed. They were, in medical terminology, paraplegic. Their upper bodies, though weakened, would probably make a full recovery, but their legs were permanently damaged and left relatively useless.

One man remains faceless in my memory. I cannot recall a single aspect of his appearance or personality. His bed was the farthest from the door, and I remember him as a chorus member, someone who laughed at the jokes but never told one, the sort of man who would respond to most suggestions, no matter what the proposal, with a "Yeah, great!"

The leader in the room occupied the center bed. He was a sly, seemingly playful man perhaps twice my age, with long straight black hair oiled and swept back over his ears. He had a narrow face with a sharp nose, which he kept pointed toward achieving his overriding ambition—a furlough and a weekend visit to his hometown on the western border of Missouri. I suppose he wanted to see his children and other members of his family. I suppose he wanted to be free of the hospital to visit his barber or to eat at his favorite restaurant. But the single ambition he expressed aloud—his primary topic of conversation—was his intent to persuade his wife into their bedroom and onto their bed so that there he might demonstrate he remained capable of sexual intercourse.

And that he did. He begged a furlough from his physician, got it, accomplished his goal with the apparent cooperation of his wife, and then returned to relay her report of his prowess.

I was interested. I was envious. I had no wife. In fact, I had no girlfriend who cared to visit more than once.

And so it went. I would tire of television or books—from Faulkner to Steinbeck and then to odd little westerns or adventure stories nameless in my memory—and I would persuade an orderly to move me into the hallway so that I might visit with passersby. And at least once a day, I would ask someone to roll my chair down to the ward. There the conversation invariably focused on sex, sports, food, the nurses, and what we were going to do when we were released.

I can call up the face of the third man in the ward, Barlow, the last among equals, most clearly. He was nineteen, but his pre-polio world had been circumscribed by his farm-boy life and his limited intellect. Among us, he was the least damaged by the disease. He had the broad sloping shoulders and powerful arms of a man who had been set to physical labor as a child. His face was pockmarked, topped by a poorly-trimmed head of dishwater-colored hair, and he perpetually wore an odd open-mouthed expression distinguished by a ragged overbite. He liked to talk, but he had little interesting or different to say, focusing instead on the gnarly obsessions and scatological interests of pre-adolescence.

One day, out of boredom and directly from the catalog of his primary preoccupation, the man who had journeyed home and satisfied his libido decided to convince Barlow that the single hope for freedom for any male patient in the polio ward resided in his ability to achieve an erection.

"These people ain't gonna let you out of here 'til you prove you ain't damaged as a man," he told Barlow.

"Yep, first time you get a stiffy you gotta call one of them nurses and tell . . ." said the chorus member.

"No, that ain't gonna do it," said the instigator. "You gotta show them. Just say, 'Lookie here. I got one. I can go now.' And pull back your cover and show 'em your hard little pecker."

And one evening as the student nurses were helping to pass out dinner trays, Barlow did just that. Whether he flipped back his blanket and said, "I'm ready to go now," I don't know. He wasn't particularly articulate. He may have simply raised the cover and said, "Look!" I only heard about the incident later. I can't remember anyone being upset, I suppose because the staff knew Barlow was Barlow and simply incapable of refined behavior.

But I had a secret. I believed Barlow instinctively understood something elemental about polio as a disease, about being an energetic young man crippled down into paralysis. Barlow understood what it had done to him, and how he would live out its consequences. His simple genius, nurtured by a lifetime of comprehending the difference between steer and bull, stud and gelding, between the independence of manhood and the lurking dependence of disability, was truer than those who played him for a fool.

The night of Barlow's conquest I thought about my own journey in the iron lung, crawling up out of the fever and delusions of polio, coming awake in the dawn of one morning, and then another, still alive, and another—thinking, then speaking, and finally feeling the initial stirrings of my nervous system attempting to reconnect its circuits. First, awkwardly, tentatively, I could move my head from side to side, and then I could flex my left hand and bend my arm slightly at the elbow, raising it up from flat beside me to fall upon my belly. And then one morning, like millions of other young males, I began to experience the surges of morning tumescence. And it hurt like the very devil, as if my penis were being yanked, stretched by being attached to a hot clamp, this reawakening of man's elemental part, that link between cell and survival, that part that strives to create.

Every day I had remained locked in the iron lung, I felt the ache burning, throbbing—a painful flowing of blood and engorging of flesh. I could not breathe, but life would not die.

And I was happy at this seeming return to . . . what? Not normalcy. Manhood, perhaps. His penis equals all things sexual to a seventeen-year-old male, of course. But set that young man's body afire with poliomyelitis and cram it in an iron lung, and the penis begins to matter not at all. Make an adolescent male sick to death, and he will burn down to asexuality. Temporarily, at least.

Somewhere in the spinning confusion before I was put into that lifesaving can, I remember a technician had wielded a urinary catheter. It was day one, or night one, of my journey, and the doctors were watching while polio decided what it was going to do to me. No matter. I was already trapped in a place where I could not void my bladder, trapped in a blurry kaleidoscope of delusions, trapped and full of pain, full of the urge and inability to urinate. It was a male technician who had arrived to insert the catheter. This was the Eisenhower era, when nurses were female and doctors generally male. Gender neutrality was evident only lower down the scale among the first-line caregivers, aides, and orderlies.

I suppose he was an orderly. I suppose he laughed inside when I grunted, "Like hell you are" after he had told me his orders.

Days later—a week or more?—the catheter no longer necessary because I was lucid, and with nurses and female aides regularly helping me use the urinal, I marveled as I moved past embarrassment and self-consciousness; I found myself fascinated that the thing that had grown to such importance as I stumbled through puberty could be handled so casually by a grown woman. I was seventeen, and it was the first time a woman other than my mother or grandmother had touched my penis.

You don't need to flip too many pages in the book of titillating fantasies to find stories featuring buxom nurses in crisp white uniforms, but, in reality, the nurses on the polio ward, while totally feminine, were so businesslike, so focused on the mechanics of care, as to seem totally sexless.

And so in that winter of my disability, as my adolescent body began its reach toward whatever normalcy it could recover and I began brandishing spontaneous and unavoidable morning erections, the nurses and female aides would thrust the urinal through one of the iron lung's portholes and say, "Here. Hold tight. Don't spill it. Yell when you're finished."

Lost in the confusion of disease, penis perceived as disposal tube rather than instrument of procreation and pleasure, I did not understand the quixotic manner in which nature reordered itself, at least not until I ventured into the ward and met the man who burned to bed his wife. Instinct conquers. Life burns, bubbles, and boils. That man knew it. He thought to teach Barlow, but the farm boy already understood the lesson. I would learn it.

10

It took the hospital administration two more months to decide how—and where—to dismiss me. I was too old to be admitted to the Shriners Crippled Children's Hospital in St. Louis, but, working with the March of Dimes, the doctors learned I could be transferred to that national organization's Rehabilitation Clinic at Creighton University Medical Center in Omaha, Nebraska. My parents were asked to find a way to get me there, and the simplest seemed to be a private air ambulance. Money was short, but somehow—with the aid of a precious $600 gathered through a community fund-raiser in Hurley—they managed. That $600 doesn't seem like much today, but it represented six dollars from every resident of the little town, and that during a period when a dollar might be the pay for six hours of labor.

Luckily, I had recovered enough strength to be able to breathe unassisted for short periods, mostly because the therapists and nurses forced me to shut off the respiratory chest shell or the rocking bed for ever-increasing periods. I would be unhooked from the chest shell, loaded on a gurney, and a technician from the physical therapy department would push me to the elevator to the basement where a whirlpool bath was located. I made these trips without using any mechanical respirator, the gurney most often powered by a man about forty or so who had cerebral palsy and moved with an odd gait. The ride was smooth enough, the fellow was always cheerful and supportive, and soon minutes away from respiratory assistance stretched to an hour or more. The prevailing idea then among those treating people who had had polio was to wean them from a respirator as soon as possible. I swung between anticipation, frustration, and panic, all without provocation or reason. No one at Burge Hospital in Springfield provided counseling during the process. No one seemed to understand the psychological influence of being unable to breathe correctly, adequately—the feeling of hysteria that pressed me down into a strange claustrophobic terror. And no one there, or at the rehabilitation center, ever checked blood gas levels or oxygen saturation to make certain patients were ventilating properly. I suppose the tests weren't available then.

In spite of the assumption that I would be able to make the flight to Omaha without a respirator, my parents hired a respiratory technician to accompany me. Two seats were removed from a little single-engine Cessna 172, and I was to be loaded on a stretcher which would be strapped down in their place. The flight would last about two hours. I was surprised to learn on the day of the flight that it was Ray, the technician who had presided over my first vital lesson in disability, who would accompany me. His means of keeping me alive if I collapsed into respiratory distress would be a hand-squeezed air bladder and a nasal mask.

I suppose with the little plane being a four-seater there was no chance for him to wander off and leave me without positive pressure. I made it to Omaha alive.

In my first days at Creighton's rehabilitation center, the doctors decided to exchange the chest shell for a pneumatic waist belt. Air pressure inflates the belt, about eight inches wide, at normal respiratory rates. The constriction of the midsection squeezes air from lungs; the relaxation of the pressure creates the vacuum that allows them to re-inflate.

Simple brute force. Squeeze hard. Guts mash air out of the lungs. Let go. Guts drop. Lungs expand. The device was less cumbersome than the chest shell. I was able to move around more, to bend and reach, and even to see my feet while I was erect in a wheelchair.

All the respiratory devices, nevertheless, carried the flaw of being mechanical not-me's. All were lifelines tossed to me while I learned to swim in the ocean of disability. All were gadgets that imposed their will upon me in the name of service.

God bless them, one and all.

While I wore the belt, and that was for a year or more, I dared not overeat. I dared not wait too long to empty my bladder.

I sweat, burn, and chafe where it rubs me. It constricts. I react.

It took but a few days before I found myself grateful for this odd and slightly violent process. It was one beat closer to normal respiratory function. My nose, mouth, lungs, and chest were free. If a stranger were to talk to me on a telephone, he might only realize I was machine-dependent because my speech patterns continued to follow the rhythm of a machine.

The weaning continued in the Omaha center. I soon found myself spending time each day free of the belt. Two of the lead doctors encouraged me to concentrate on breathing using what remained of my diaphragm muscles.

"Watch that. Don't use your neck muscles or your stomach muscles. Diaphragm. Diaphragm."

Another physician, a woman trained in Hungary, a refugee who had fled from the darkness behind the Iron Curtain to the open skies of the Great Plains, hinted that I should ignore them. Dr. Antal was small, somewhat careworn, a few inches over five feet. As I sat in the wheelchair, the top of my head reached her nose. She had an edgy face, intelligent eyes, beautiful dark brown hair shot with silver.

"Breathe however," she said. "Breathe. No matter. More breathing on your own, less machines. Neck muscles are fine. Stomach muscles good. Just breathe."

Years later, when I saw the famous Dr. Elisabeth Kubler-Ross speaking on television, this female doctor came to mind. My doctor's appearance and mannerisms were very much similar to the famous author of *On Death and Dying*.

But Dr. Antal's specialty was living.

At least, that's the attention she directed toward me. As withdrawn, unaware, and insensitive as I was then, I think now that she was somewhat a maverick within the clinic. She roamed the wards and hallways alone. The other physicians were trailed by nurses and orderlies. She looked each patient in the eye and addressed each one directly. She touched us.

Dr. Antal would lean toward me as she spoke, as if being as near as possible to me might compensate for her unfamiliarity with English grammar and syntax. She wanted to teach me the technique of frog-breathing, an essential skill for anyone with no cough reflex, something I had seen Keith take to naturally, but something I had never attempted. I caught on to the technique immediately. None of the other doctors had mentioned its importance, but she seemed a realist, recognizing pain and frustration and fear and the necessity of coping in any way possible.

The other doctors, no doubt having cultivated a useful detachment which allowed them to function ankle-deep in pain and death, came across as mechanics of the human body. Dr. Antal had mastered the ability to see the person without ignoring the illness or injury. I think she believed in people; the other physicians believed in technology. I think she believed that a good life, a happy life, is made up of the pieces of circumstance and scraps of random luck that come our way, and it's up to us to build a suitable place to live that life.

And I think she liked it that I listened when she talked.

Charlie, a college student working as an orderly, had been my guide when I first arrived at the Creighton Clinic. Many of the other staff at the clinic were also students at the Jesuit-run university.

Charlie initially seemed a friendly sort, popular with both staff and patients, someone only a few years older with whom I might connect. He pushed me through the halls and into some of the offices, introducing me to staff and patients. And with us went Charlie's favorite companion, a middle-age man recuperating from a severe head injury. According to the story I would soon learn, the man had been seriously injured in an auto accident. He had recovered physically, but his demeanor and his mental capacity had reverted to childlike levels. The rumor also said he would progress no further.

The old man trailed the young orderly constantly, shuffling along in khakis, a long-sleeve shirt, and slippers. The supervisors accepted the man's constant desire to follow Charlie during his duties. The man seldom spoke, but he would cheerfully take on simple chores like carrying clean linens as beds were changed. The only drawback, ward rumor had it, was that he could randomly descend into fits of rage.

I lived at the center for three months, and nearly every time I saw the tall, thin, blond-headed orderly, the old man with a white crewcut would be bobbing along peacefully in his wake. One of the nurses told me the old man had been a prominent commercial artist, his crowning achievement the design of a logo for a beer can. The gossipers were sure it was Falstaff. It was a good story, one we eagerly related to every new face.

Creighton was a Catholic institution, with a padre making the rounds once a week or so, paying attention mostly to his fellow believers; we saw the nuns who apparently administered the hospital slightly more often. And compared to Burge Hospital in Springfield, I noticed there were far more male orderlies than female aides, the people we patients interacted with most often. That left the nurses to supervise the staff and allowed the doctors to march through on their parade of daily rounds and then disappear.

I noticed two or three young Native Americans, Lakotas, I think, and two foreigners—all of them students—but my favorite among the orderlies was Clint. I think he perceived me as something other than a nasty set of chores. About forty, Clint had a spare frame, a laborer's hands, and a receding hairline slicked back with Wildroot Cream Oil. He was the quietest of the bunch. I was intrigued by the expression in his eyes, which swung between boredom, confusion, and amusement. During the afternoon as things slowed down, he would come into my part of the ward smelling of peppermint schnapps and pull a chair up near my bed. Together Clint and I would watch the daily feature race from Ak-Sar-Ben, the horse-racing track in Omaha. I would tell him stories about my Uncle Charlie and his race horses, and he would tell me stories about not being able to pick a winner.

I could understand the schnapps. The guy was the only one for whom working as an orderly was a permanent job. I remember nothing of Clint's life outside the ward. I don't think he was married, and he was always willing to pull an extra shift. The rest of the group were time-servers, earning the money necessary to sustain themselves while they prepared for something better.

I was comfortable with my schnapps-drinking friend, and Clint seemed to gravitate toward me because I liked to talk about the ponies. If I asked for help, Clint seemed always amenable. On the other hand, like most people turned totally dependent, I also began to weed out those who required careful handling.

And with a few, there were always hints that we crips were at their mercy. It's a nasty thing to contemplate, I know, but the smartest crip soon appreciates that dependency—the appearance of helplessness—can open a door to a dark room in some psyches.

Surprisingly, it turned out that Charlie, the college student I first thought friendly, was one I learned to watch warily. Like many young men, Charlie was boisterous and sometimes rough, but the situation could reach a flash point. That happened most often when he worked with one of the enlisted men who earned a few extra dollars at the center when not on duty at the local Air Force base. Nearly every time they landed on the same shift, the two seemed to pull some sort of prank. Shamefully, I was still a callow teenager, and I occasionally found myself amused by some of their escapades. I also wanted to avoid being a target. I knew instinctively if I joined in, which in my case meant laughter or approving comments, I didn't need to protect myself—a playground lesson that came in handy now that I couldn't run away.

11

Other than the orderlies, the two staff members I saw most were the physical therapist and the occupational therapist, the latter a profession I never knew existed before I went to Omaha.

Physical therapy was easy. I had the use of my hands and a majority of the muscles in my arms. I could wiggle my left leg, tense and relax the few muscles left undamaged there, but the leg would not support sufficient weight to allow me to be fitted with braces. My right leg was even weaker.

No treadmills. No sweat. Other than a rubber ball to squeeze and develop hand strength, plus a five-pound weight for my arms, I was worked on rather than told to work out. The faceless, disinterested therapists concentrated on flexing my ankles, knees, and hips to extend my range of motion. Leg folded, knee to chest; leg extended, ankle over belly-button. Twenty-five repetitions. Maybe I would never be able to move my legs, but they were intent making it possible for someone else to fold me up and put me away if necessary.

I had been a reluctant participant in my recovery process at Burge Hospital. Most of the exercises there had focused on getting me out of the iron lung and into a wheelchair. Burge had physical therapists but no rehabilitation specialists. After attempts to flex and stretch my muscles, and whirlpool baths to soothe them, I think the doctors and therapists understood I would never be strong enough to stand with braces or walk with crutches. Better that I become someone else's problem.

That meant there was a price to pay when I got to Omaha. Therapy hurt, near torture in my self-involved adolescent imagination.

But three or four times a week, they laid hands on me and cranked out a few more grudging degrees of ankle, knee, and hip movement each session. No massages beforehand; no rub-downs after. Simply stretches and more stretches.

I was a bungled job, and the silent, white-clad automatons were the clean-up crew. They only talked to complain about the results of neglected treatment in Springfield. I moaned, groaned, and whimpered, attempting to endure the pain. I may as well have stayed silent.

My joints were almost locked. My muscles had atrophied, and it seemed every nerve resided at skin-level. Worse, the mess I had made of my body by complaining and resisting every attempt at rigorous therapy in Springfield was severely aggravated by five pressure sores, the result of not being turned regularly while in the iron lung.

The decubitus ulcer on my hip had eaten the flesh nearly to my tailbone. Those on my elbows had begun to close after I moved to the rocking bed and wheelchair, but the ones on my heels remained open, weeping and bleeding, because I could not move my legs while sleeping. Those four, one each on elbows and heels, were easy to attack. The fact that I used a wheelchair a good part of each day at the center resulted in more freedom from damaging pressure, and the therapists rigged up a set of foam braces to elevate my heels during the night. But the one located at the base of my spine remained an open wound. That meant my physical therapy routine consisted of manipulation, highlighted by burning pain inflicted on joints that I swore would crack; time in a whirlpool, with me unable to hide my fear of drowning because I could no longer swim; and then several minutes under an ultraviolet light after my ulcerated wound was bathed in common vinegar.

Physical therapy consumed a good part of the day, and occupational therapy most of the remainder. The two were separated by lunch, and I traveled between these stations of rehabilitation pushed along by an attendant.

What purpose OT was to serve me, I never understood. If the damage evident was to be damage permanent, I should have been trained to do something with my brains rather than my hands. The therapist was a friendly, open-faced guy with a blond crew cut. He was the sort who used artificial enthusiasm and constant cheerfulness to establish distance from the patients and thereby keep control of the situation. There was a typewriter in the OT room, and that made some sense to me, but I didn't comprehend the purpose of by-the-number paint sets or leather-working kits. I understood and liked words, and so I gravitated to the typewriter and banged away happily, mostly writing nonsense when I wasn't writing a letter home. I thought the other activities best suited for kindergarten. Leather was for cowboy boots and belts to support big buckles. As for art, I appreciated Goya, Van Gogh, and Norman Rockwell, none of whom painted by number.

I soon learned occupational therapy, a misnomer to a naïve observer like me, was more about developing physical dexterity and providing a sense of accomplishment than it was about preparing anyone to earn a living. In fact, during the entire time at the Omaha rehabilitation center, no one asked me, "What would you like to do with your life? How do you plan on earning a living?"

I wish they had. Better said, I wish I had known the question needed to be asked. Rich or poor, whole or damaged, we are responsible for ourselves.

This was 1960, and the subtext of every interaction between patient and staff was to teach the patient how to cope with the effects of a disability, which as far as I could observe there in the center consisted mostly of severe conditions with minimal hope for improvement. This was 1960, and the lack of sophisticated assistive devices, and the closed-off attitudes of both the public and the medical professionals, meant reintegration into society ended at almost the same point it had since catastrophic injury and illness became survivable.

You're crippled. You're going to be crippled the remainder of your life. This is how to put on a shirt. This is how to pee in a urinal while sitting in a wheelchair. Here, when you're finished, you can make a leather wallet to keep busy until it's time for your favorite television show.

No one expressed any idea that it might be preferable—or even possible—to train and educate people with disabilities so that they could function as productive workers and professionals in society. No one said, "Some sort of disability, some sort of disadvantage, visible or invisible, is part of the human condition. Live fully with yours as you see it. Be assured others do as well with their own perceived disability, visible or not."

The lesson I needed then should have been stated bluntly. *You are a cripple. You will never walk again. You will be dependent on the care of others. Cry and complain for a while if you like. That's normal. Then we will help you find something useful to do with your life.*

Granted, there was an overriding passion at the center for compensation through technology. Wheelchairs, special beds, crutches, and leg braces, of course, were sensible enough for those who needed them, but no one said outright, "This will be the key element in finding you a job." They were provided simply for mobility and comfort. On the other hand, there were a number of devices that seemed to have no advantages at all. For example, one of the keys to my success in moving about the world, the occupational therapist seemed to think, would be braces for my hands and load-bearing platforms for my arms.

The hand braces, once custom-built, looked like brass knuckles with a thumb rack. They weren't brass, of course. They were aluminum with padded inserts and a leather strap to buckle them securely. The thumb rack was meant to hold my polio thumb in "normal" position—that is, less flat like a monkey's digit and more in opposition like a human being's.

Polio is an odd disease, sometimes fatal but always fickle. It's fickle because the virus destroys nerve paths, hit and miss. Some people are paralyzed in one limb, some in two, some in more, but if it affects a person's upper body it often eats up the nerve path to the muscle which gives the hand an opposable thumb. The muscle atrophies and the thumb thereafter lays flat, like a monkey's. To emphasize its whimsical nature, the disease can leave the rest of the fingers on the hand relatively undamaged.

When I'm out in public, or when I watch television, I sometimes still catch a glimpse of a polio thumb. Actually, poliomyelitis is all but dead in the developed world, and so when I see them they mostly decorate the hands of people my age or older.

The OT ideal, as I remember, was to wear the special braces to train my hands to stay in a proper position. To eat, to hold a pen or pencil, or to do anything else requiring a firm grip, I had to remove the braces. That meant I couldn't wear them most of the time. And so, after I got home, I showed them to my father, a friend or two, and then tossed them in a drawer.

Next came the load-bearing platforms for my arms. The array of muscles along my back and much of my shoulders were generally useless. I couldn't then or now sit in my wheelchair and lift my arms over my head, for example. The therapist decided more natural arm movement could be imitated by building two metal units to mount on the uprights framing the back of my wheelchair. Where the gadgets bolted onto the chair back, there were horizontal "shoulder" bearings. Midway down each device, there was an "elbow" bearing. I could pick up one arm up with the other, lay it in the rack, and have a full range of shoulder and elbow movement, except for raising my hands over my head, which was the thing I needed most to do. The only problem was that I had to take my arms out of the racks to roll my wheelchair, and, once free, the racks had a tendency to flop around and get hung on door jambs or in other tight spaces.

All this occupational and physical therapy was carried out under a doctor's prescription, of course, but I cannot remember seeing any physician during the sessions. In fact, as far as the center was concerned, I was a child, a minor with no control over my course of treatment; it had been mapped out in a brief conference with my mother, who had taken the bus from Springfield to Omaha the day after I was admitted. I had no authority to consent to the implementation of any treatment. I accepted that. I had been a youngster before I got polio, a teenager living under my parents' roof and dependent upon their support, and so there was no reason for me to believe adults lacked authority over me in Omaha.

Age seventeen was the wrong time to become a cripple, at least for me. I had begun to recognize that my father's rigid attitudes and authoritarian manner did not represent the world in which I wanted to live. He was in control of his life. I wanted to be in control of mine, but I had not completely charted my path to that position.

Now I found myself nearly helpless—reduced to voicing complaints but incapable of taking action—and subject to the control of other people. I could not transfer from bed to wheelchair or wheelchair to bed without assistance. I could find a urinal and empty my bladder, but I needed help before I could attempt a bowel movement. I could slip on a shirt, if someone would reach into a closet and get it for me, but I could not put on my shoes, socks, or a pair of pants. Lay me on a bed, and I was as helpless as a box turtle flipped on its back.

And so the physicians decided, my parents concurred, and I received.

Or rather, my mother concurred after consulting with my father. He was tied to the farm, every dollar of his savings invested in the land and in a small herd of dairy cows. Dairy cows cannot be left unmilked, and he had no money to hire someone to do the job for him. There also was the question of my brother, Jon. We had no family nearby, no trusted close friends, with whom Jon could stay if my father wanted to drive to Omaha. My father and Jon had been able to visit regularly while I was hospitalized in Springfield, an hour's drive from our place, but now he could not afford the time or the money to journey to Omaha.

It did not matter to me, really. I was content to be a momma's boy. Since my father had been caught up in World War II during the first years of my life, I suppose it took me far longer than the average child to develop the fundamental comprehension of the three of us as a family. If I wanted something, I relied on my mother. In fact, I had been an only child until I was nearly nine and the only grandchild on my mother's side for almost as long. The family's little prince, I loved, relied upon, and subconsciously manipulated my mother, my aunt, and my maternal grandparents, the people with whom I spent a good part of my first five or six years. I had no doubt my father loved me, but he knew of only one way to accomplish anything and that was through courage and perseverance. Nursing—nurturing—was women's work, and it took a kind of bravery he might have known that he didn't have.

I believed my father would have visited Omaha, if possible, but even if the cows were only an excuse, I understood. And accepted. But the doctor in charge of the clinic, a pot-bellied middle-aged fellow with a receding hairline and a three-piece suit, couldn't tolerate my father's absence and became frustrated. He wanted my father there to receive the pronouncements handed down for my treatment.

If the doctor relied on the idea that a man's place was to make decisions and act on behalf of his family, he'd never met an army wife, my mother in particular. She was soft and sweet. And strong. She had traveled alone to Europe and Asia with me in tow, and she had moved her household by herself several other times. She took control during each of her visits. The doctor had age and authority on his side, but not passion. I was her son, and to deal with me, he must first deal with her.

Despite the veneer of sophistication painted on by years of city living and world travel, my parents were people of a make-do, tolerate-discomfort culture, the Anglo-Celt descendants of the hardscrabble hill country Appalachian population. They expected no favors or sympathy, and I was to stand straight and take the same attitude. The description fit my father most of all, and I envied his toughness, his grit, his stoicism, his ability to be too cold or too hot or too wounded and yet carry on. After I found myself in the iron lung, I felt I should apologize to him for my failure, for my physical weakness, for becoming forever dependent.

Even now, I grieve for his soul's despair as his firstborn—not me, but rather his child, his idea of me—fell into paralysis and never got up again.

He was a strong man, my father, but sometimes strength isn't enough. And most of all, somewhere deep inside me, I knew he believed it was often best to shoot the wounded and bury the pain.

I did too, at least within the part of me that did not fear oblivion.

12

Looking back, I realize my sojourn at the center, at that putative training ground for crips, was the only time during my life on wheels that I have been totally immersed in the milieu of the permanently banged-up and battered. It was a window into a world I had never imagined.

One guy in his early twenties was there for a tune-up, exactly why I don't remember. Crips can be prone to pressure sores, kidney stones, and other maladies. Like me, he was from Missouri. He smoked, so badly addicted that he had an ash tray welded to one arm of his wheelchair. His ambition was to be a jeweler. He had a flat face highlighted by a sharp nose and light brown hair, talked with a twang, and nearly always kept one eye in a permanent squint from the cigarette smoke.

Another guy a few years older than me had been pulled from under a toppled piece of construction equipment and then racked up in a Stryker frame to allow his broken spine to heal. I was fascinated by the huge device, made of parallel stainless steel hoops perhaps ten feet in diameter. Between the hoops, a bed frame was mounted on bearings, and the patient could be strapped in, braced, and then rotated 360 degrees on both the vertical and horizontal axes. The idea was to change the patient's position regularly to avoid pressure sores, pneumonia, and other maladies.

I saw the guy, said hello, and we exchanged war stories. After a few words, I noticed he was distracted. Most of his attention was focused on keeping his wife from collapsing into a permanent state of panic. She was obviously overwhelmed with the injury to her young husband and uncomfortable with the place where it had left him—the rehabilitation center, that great impersonal building filled with the maimed and mangled. A woman in her early twenties should be thinking of babies and her first house rather than visiting her husband while he's strapped to a device resembling something out of a medieval dungeon.

The guy I talked with most, other than the orderly who liked peppermint schnapps and horse-racing, was a city police officer recuperating from a gunshot wound. He had a private room, no doubt courtesy of the city. The cop had pale Scandinavian blond hair and a cynical grin. His wife was the same Nordic type, and she and his cotton-topped kids apparently visited him daily. The story was that he'd been part of a group of officers who chased a bad guy from Omaha across the Missouri River and into Council Bluffs, Iowa. The cops had cornered the fugitive in a house, and there had been a shoot-out. This cop had taken a bullet through the neck, and it had damaged his spinal cord in a bizarre fashion. Both legs and his right arm were totally paralyzed while his left arm remained completely functional.

I envied him the power of that arm. At that point, I could move my hands, my forearms, and a few other muscles, but I was weak, hardly able to lift five-pound weights. He could accomplish more with his single working arm than I could with both hands.

I also envied his more glamorous story, a heroic tale of gunfire and bloodshed so much more romantic than a failed inoculation. I heard the story several times, first when he told it to me, and later when I was nearby as he regaled other visitors. I would laugh with him when he came to the part where he described lying wounded on the ground and unable to move, all the while screaming, "Shoot the son of a bitch! Shoot him! Shoot him!" I suppose the other cops did, although I don't remember the guy ever saying so directly.

The cop's room was decorated with flowers and cards, plus a number of personal items like a console television. No doubt that was a gift of a grateful city. He also scooted around the halls of the center in a power wheelchair, a crip Cadillac so to speak. He had more visitors than any other patient, and so those of us who weren't heroes served mostly as a crip chorus.

As I integrated myself into the center's milieu, I discovered I was scheduled for visits with the staff psychological therapist. On my first visit, I learned the man had been a bomber navigator during World War II, flying combat missions over occupied Europe. That history contrasted with his mellow manner and tweedy appearance—tie and vest over rotund belly, the approach of middle-age evident in receding wavy hair. I thought about the cop and his *Shoot the SOB!* story, and I wondered what the therapist had said in response when the cop had told him.

I think I was sent—pushed—to the shrink's office sometime during the first weeks of my stay. Maybe it was one of the first stops for every newly admitted crip. That made sense to me. I instinctively wanted someone to talk to who cared about more than my momentary physical needs. I had an inkling that my predicament was going to take more guts than I had, but I was too ignorant and unsophisticated to realize someone should have been doctoring my head long before I landed in Omaha.

Most of the talk up to that point had been about "improving my attitude," a phrase I had heard long before I ended up in the hospital. My mother had babied me most of my life, but my father had never let me use the word "can't." By the time I was drafted into the crip army, I was a quiet, spoiled, and often resentful kid who coped with tough situations by being nagged into persistence, with failure by relying on petulance, and with denial by sneaking around to do what I wanted.

And I was a dreamer, someone too willing to think *If only* . . . rather than develop a plan and work to achieve a goal. Looking back, it's obvious my personality incorporated at least half a dozen attributes a good crip needs the least.

I knew I could use help, but my initial visit with the psychologist left me confused. I didn't think I was crazy, but I hadn't thought I would get polio either. Now I believed I needed to listen to new ideas about how to cope. Nevertheless, I probably only subconsciously comprehended I really was going to have my ass planted in a wheelchair for a long time. What I needed was straight talk, goals to focus on, and means to reach them. What I needed was someone to say, "The picture you had of your future has been erased. This mess you're in is real, and you're going to need to assemble another future out of the broken parts."

The initial visit, however, wasn't about crazy or not crazy or depression and coping. It was, as far as I could understand, about determining the level of my intelligence.

At that point, I may have been smart enough to understand that smart wasn't going to get me out of a wheelchair, but I wasn't smart enough to realize what that meant. Yes, smart enough to comprehend that I would be crippled beyond movement—crippled, in fact, both in attitude and opportunity—but life would be hell on wheels until I grew smart enough to understand the wheelchair was irrelevant to happiness.

The psychologist asked, "Can you name four U.S. presidents who have served in the twentieth century?"

"Hmm, let's see. How about Eisenhower, Truman, FDR, and Hoover?" I wondered if I would receive extra points for naming them in reverse order.

Even though I would have liked to have made regular visits, I saw the shrink only one or two more times. I learned something I already knew: my IQ wasn't paralyzed. Actually, I had wanted to go more often, but apparently as bright as I thought myself I wasn't bright enough to earn regular visits by crying, refusing to eat, or indulging irrational anger.

I know now I would have been best served by an empathetic, supportive listener who offered a practical response to permanent paralysis. I know now what I really wanted was sympathy for my predicament and reassurance that everything was going to be all right.

But there was another reason I wanted to make regular visits to the shrink's office, equally self-interested but not as important. I liked his secretary. She was only a few years older than me, and also polio-wounded like me, but she was only paralyzed from the waist down. I thought she was quite attractive, with brunette hair, a clear complexion, and a generous bosom. She was a graceful young woman, feminine in her movements, dancing behind her desk with her still legs invisible.

I know she felt me following her with my eyes, even though I was too shy to push any conversation past the "How are you" stage. I suppose she liked the attention, but I suspect she considered me simply one more crip moving down the rehab reassembly line and thus not worth any investment of emotional energy.

Later in my stay at the rehab center, one of the aides told me the young woman lived at the hospital. She earned her keep by working on the staff. A good enough arrangement, I thought, without relating it to my situation. My IQ may have been undamaged—I could have told the shrink that Coolidge came before Hoover and Harding before Coolidge if he needed more proof—but even that information didn't provide me with a solid grip on the idea that I too would have to live out the rest of my life as something other than a victim of polio.

I stayed at the rehabilitation center from February 1960 to May 1960, turning eighteen in the process. I left completely ignorant of how to cope with this thing I had become. I left not because the experts were done with me but because the March of Dimes unit that financed my stay had run out of money.

My mother rode up to Omaha on the bus again so that she could fly home with me. The orderlies wished me good luck and helped my mother pack my stuff. As we left, we met the head of the clinic, still dressed in his traditional three-piece suit and lab coat. He had a set of instructions for my mother, things like a special diet to avoid kidney stones and the name of a free clinic for crippled children in Springfield.

He held onto my arm after we shook hands, and he rotated my wrist so that he had a clear view of my polio thumb.

"When he comes back," he said, looking at my mother, "we can operate to move the tendon from his ring finger over to his thumb, replacing the atrophied muscle. He'll have a normal grip."

I looked at my mother, and she looked at me. Neither of us said anything.

13

And so, the experts supposedly having done their best, my mother and I journeyed home in another little Cessna four-seater, sailing down off the Great Plains into the Ozark hills, there to begin a life neither of us knew how to live.

What I remember most about that flight was landing in Springfield. The door to the airplane opened, and Dad reached toward the stretcher on which I rode, grasped my hand, and said, "How are you, son?"

I was proud that I didn't cry.

The pilot helped my father transfer me out of the airplane and into our car. We drove the thirty-five miles southwest to our farm with me propped up at an angle in the rear seat. The flight and the quick trip home consumed nearly all the precious hours I could then tolerate without respirator assistance. It was a green spring season, and, even though I had only spent a few months in Missouri before polio hit, I found landmarks that were familiar—the arrow-straight road leading south from U.S. Highway 60, bordered for miles by prosperous dairy farms, then the steep drop as we turned toward Spring Creek valley and the abandoned mill at Hurley.

That journey from the rehabilitation center to the little rock house a mile from Spring Creek was the reordering of a family life, after which my parents became physically what I had lost, when my mother and father began to function where I could not, to accomplish everything from wiping the feces from my rectum and lifting my body out of bed, to tending to my needs of the day and then returning me to bed.

As all the equipment necessary to sustain me was unloaded at our farm house, my brother Jon confronted the new and disabled reality of our family. The rocking bed itself consumed almost half the space of the small bedroom we had shared. Jon took up residence in our former back porch, which my father had enclosed and insulated so that it might serve as a small bedroom.

Our family had been attacked by a virus and exploded, leaving Jon, only eight years old, a sometimes forgotten bystander. Nearly every older sibling will live to reconcile guilt over failures in brother-or-sisterhood, of course. I know I could have been a better, more loving brother before I became a crip, and after as well. I love my brother deeply, and as we've grown older we've begun to care for one another, to offer one another support, to understand we are all of what's left of the little family that once roamed the world from army fort to army fort.

But only now am I old enough to forget—to forgive fate—that throughout his formative years I was too busy being crippled to be a brother.

That Jon's life has not been much handicapped by my disability, at least in a practical sense, we owe to my father, a man born in 1916. In my father's experience any person using a wheelchair was an "invalid." I believe my father made a significant effort to isolate Jon from the challenges of my disability. My disability was my own, to be shared only with those first responsible for my life, my mother and father. Jon's life was his own.

Of course, at first and in truth, my father had no reason to believe that I wasn't an invalid. I acted like one after I returned home, waiting to be waited upon, more focused on limitations than possibilities. I know I was the wrong person at the wrong time and wrong place to join the crip brigade—a teenager in the rural Midwest in 1960—but I will forever harbor regrets over my failures in those years. I know there was an undercurrent of darker emotions, no doubt contrived by my own psyche. Even before my paralysis, I had the feeling that I reflected the disappointments my father found in his own life, perhaps for no other reason than that this person who resembled him so closely showed no more than average promise. His firstborn wasn't West Point material.

Paralysis became proof.

It is only right that my father wanted to make certain my brother would not be forced to drag the anchor of my disability through his life. I accepted that and gradually became an interested observer and then cheerleader in Jon's life as he worked his way through high school and college.

But it took me a long time—because of physical isolation, because society had yet to make available access for people with disabilities, and because of the I follow orders aspect of my passive personality—to learn to think independently, to grow into a brother.

I needed an attitude adjustment in other ways as well. One of the less useful results of my stay at the rehabilitation clinic was that it delayed my recognition that I had been transformed—that I was ready to be thrust out into the world as a cripple. I had yet to fully recognize that. Now, down on the farm, I sat waiting for lessons.

I don't know how long it took my parents to reconcile what had happened to them. But it took me longer than necessary—perhaps ten or fifteen years, or even twenty, to begin to come to terms with being paralyzed, and being dependent. It only began after I learned to separate the rewards of the mundane, the joys promised by every sunrise, from the despair that sometimes descended in the hours before dawn.

I had fallen ill in October, moved from Springfield to Omaha in February, and gone home in May. During all those hectic months, I don't know if the doctors in Springfield or in Omaha, or anyone else for that matter, suggested that my parents institutionalize me. I never asked. I never doubted they would care for me. I was their child.

Of course, at seventeen or eighteen, I had no conception of what would be demanded of them, of how their dreams had been shattered, of the unforeseen damage inflicted on their future. And even though my parents weren't the sort to shirk responsibilities, I think like me they were ignorant of the ramifications of the catastrophe that would collapse our family. Neither one had had a severely disabled relative in their immediate family. Neither one had been close to any families with physically disabled members.

After I was discharged from Creighton, the three of us were set down to sort out circumstances none of us chose, circumstances that required two to sacrifice to sustain one, circumstances that seemed to leave the one trapped in perpetual childhood. We needed guidance and an outside perspective. None of that was available. Ironically, given our natures, we probably wouldn't have accepted it even if it had been.

The name today for that which my parents alone did for me is "personal care attendants." In the twenty-first century, there are government bureaucracies and other support groups to provide funds to help people with disabilities hire and supervise such aides. Those programs permit a person with a disability to live independently. Such programs are not universal, though. Some less enlightened entities will warehouse potential PCA clients in nursing homes, but that's another story.

My parents cared for me, even while coping with daily chores on the dairy farm. I was never neglected, living in the presence of love and sacrifice rather than stoic submission to social pressures. I heard no complaints from them about undue obligations. Instead from my mother I heard expressions of comfort and encouragement, and from my father I heard words challenging me not to bog down in self-pity.

We talked little about their obligations. If I apologized, I heard words defining moral obligations. They offered care. I accepted it, without question but not without guilt.

Of course, when a crip is plopped down in the middle of a family, there will be enough guilt for everyone, if you want the truth. My father, I suspect, felt some guilt for choosing the wrong place and time to leave the army and retreat to his conception of a clean and simple life—a place where his child found polio instead of the demons running loose in a Texas border city at the edge of Fort Bliss.

My father had retired in late 1958, a major in the U.S. Army Reserves after more than twenty-two years on active duty. I think now he retired simply because he was tired of the army. He never acted as if he was. He always kept his shoes shined, his khakis creased, and his troops toeing the mark. He grew roses and golfed on the weekend and was present and accounted for at the fort before seven o'clock every Monday morning.

We had settled in a rock house in a rocky valley across Spring Creek from the abandoned one-room schoolhouse called Blackjack. Oaks, black walnuts, and cedars covered the hills, but the cleared slopes and the creek bottoms were rich with lespedeza, clover, and other grasses. It was there my father returned to the life he'd fled, out of the Dust Bowl, out of the Great Depression, heading for the Golden State as a young man with three friends riding in a worn-out Model T. How long it had been his dream to return again to live in the presence of animals, among people who lived with, from, and upon nature, he never said.

Nor did he voice his feelings about the nightmare of polio crippling one of his sons before the end of his first year on the land.

I would have preferred to stay in Texas, and I think my mother would have also. There she had a new home with a manicured lawn and rose gardens, time to play cards and visit with friends, and grand department stores like El Paso's White House to browse. In Missouri, she had an old house half as large, neighbors caught up in the activities of interrelated families, and three miles of dirt road to reach a little settlement with one general store.

I believe my mother carried the greatest burden of guilt over my paralysis—a helpless gut-wrenching guilt I've come to believe only a mother can feel. She feared she was the one who had begun the melancholy chain of events that left me in the iron lung. My mother had seized upon the news of Dr. Salk's miracle vaccine and rushed my brother and me to the first clinic offering the inoculations.

"Gary, honey, really. I thought it was the right thing to do," she would say.

My mother possessed a classic strong jaw line, a wide smile, and a straight nose, all lit by pale blue eyes revealing an open character.

My mother was nourishment and protection and support. She lives even now in the shadow drifting down when I close my eyes, a quiet, happy, approving spirit, understanding things I might never voice to anyone else, forgiving hurts I inflict upon myself. I treasure all that is good in me as her gift.

My mother always sought joy to fill her days, but when we spoke of the unreasonable reason for me being paralyzed her eyes would widen and then pinch down in pain.

Bright blue pain.

"Don't worry about it, Mom. I wanted the shots. I knew what polio was, what it could do, about the irons lungs and the wheelchairs and braces. I wanted the shots. It's no one's fault."

I was born guilty. Not in the Christian sense of original sin, although I am willing to admit it is there, flawed man disappointing his Creator, the omniscient One having seasoned our spiritual stew with the pepper of free will. No, I was born to feel an emotional and psychological guilt for the things I have done and the things I have failed to do. I am certain I even possess an extra twisted little gene somewhere on my DNA staircase that permits me to feel guilt for failing to live up to the expectations of other people.

Nature versus nurture, you say? True enough, but not entirely so. I am not the only child bound to fail to exceed his father's dreams of self-fulfillment, but I possessed the capacity to cook my own inadequacies into this gourmet broth of guilt because I wasn't a superb athlete or a straight-A student or a hard worker instead of a dreamer.

Petty stuff, that. Grow up. Move on. Find your own bliss.

I have done so, more or less. I stopped judging my actions according to my father's standards, a characteristic of both the immature and the mature.

But real guilt—the irrational, rational, unbearable, bearable guilt as solid as the steel frame of the wheelchair I will use the remainder of my days—descended after I returned home, crippled in body and spirit, for my parents to deal with—to wake me up, put me on the bed pan, dress me, feed me, wash me, lift me back into bed, undress me, all the while making certain the odd mechanisms sent home with me would sustain my breathing. That guilt I will carry to my grave.

For years I remained blind to all that. For years I even used my predicament to challenge the two people hurting in a way I will never comprehend.

"Do you think God wants me in this wheelchair?" I asked my father sometimes when I wanted to lash out.

"How should I know?" my father would reply.

I may have asked him because I was puzzled by the notion of being crippled, fearful of its consequences, and angry over all that seemingly was being denied me. The question even may have been a legitimate one between father and son; nevertheless, I am sorry I asked it.

Hearing it, my father must have seethed with anger because he believed he had done all the right things—had been a faithful and supportive husband and had provided generously for his sons. What frustration he must have felt, frustration beyond words, that fate had paralyzed his firstborn and sent the kid home for him to reconstruct once more. My father was a few months short of his forty-fourth birthday then, still young enough to dream and hope, and he found himself facing a future shackled to my need for physical care.

God's will, indeed.

I know my question about God's designs made me feel important. I know it was a feeble, unsophisticated attempt to shift the blame for the mess of being helpless and dependent. It was God's fault, not mine. Perhaps, ever the romantic, I thought I was ordained to roll through the remainder of my life in a wheelchair because God, for reasons too bizarre to be questioned, would anoint the madness with some sort of sanctity.

God wants me in the wheelchair—all I need to do is sit here and see what happens—free eats, television all day long, lots of books, no need to work, only wait for the revelation.

Over the years, I used the question whenever my father and I skirmished along the borders of our relationship. He did not, he could not, give me a yes or no answer, which made my inquiries both pointless and pointed. His replies always carried with them a degree of frustration, puzzlement, and anger. That I thought my father should have an answer, and should be able to make me believe it was true, illustrates something about a character warped by self-pity.

And it reveals something about us both that we might each have believed it was so, that God truly wanted me in a wheelchair.

Then what?

My mother's faith was stronger, and without fail she would answer yes, that this was God's will. It was the only way she could accept that I was going to ride out the rest of my life in the chair. But she never answered, and I tried not to ask, the logical next question: "Why?"

I was closer emotionally to my mother, this woman who had received her newly crippled son home shortly before her fortieth birthday. I recognized she had steel in her—I had seen it—but I knew she had to be terribly afraid or badly hurt before you could find it. I did not want to be a cause of such a wound, at least not deliberately, not with the question of "Why?"

My father, I thought foolishly, was all steel. He was given to monosyllabic answers and to repeating unanswerable questions in different words to shift the burden of the indecipherable, to ignore the ramifications of the question, to challenge the questioner to think for himself. With him, I persisted, never failing to believe eventually he would give me the answer I wanted.

But I never knew what that answer might be.

Ah, guilt. Unspoken guilt. Helpless guilt. Useless guilt. If you want to speak of guilt, I can move forward and describe the complicated whirlpool of emotions swirling between a dying woman and her quadriplegic adult son, the son she brought from love onto this earth, the son who went willingly at her direction to accept the thing that would leave him . . . paralyzed, dependent forever.

The son, grown into a man who believed he had sucked from his mother the time and energy that she rightfully should have devoted to her own happiness.

She died, and she rests where there is no burden of guilt to carry.

But the sorry story does not end there. My father followed my mother into eternity only a year later. Never in our forty-six years together was a word about guilt exchanged between us. The guilt lies in this.

A hundred times I asked him, "Do you think God wants me in this wheelchair?"

The best he could do was to reply, "How should I know? Maybe. You're there, aren't you?"

I forgive him for having no answer.

I want to forgive myself for asking.

14

When my father retired from the army and decided to move to Missouri, we left an ethnically diverse city and moved into a culture where religion was the hard rock foundation of a hill country rural society. Sunday morning sermons were followed by Sunday night meetings and Wednesday evening prayer services. Religion was salvation promised, of course, but it was also a significant part of the social life of the community. People less impressed with the mystical might say it also provided enough passionate theater to serve as entertainment.

We weren't church people, which our neighbors found odd. My mother had been raised in a church and would have preferred to attend, but she wouldn't go alone. I think she felt the call of normalcy, of community within worship, and she bore a natural appreciation of the grace of a life lived in praise and joy, and the reassurance of unquestioned belief in a Creator who held His universe in the palm of His hand. She refused to attend church by herself, I think, not out of martyrdom but rather out of loyalty, the desire not to separate herself from her husband. My father would visit a church for a wedding or a funeral, and he sang "The Old Rugged Cross" and "Peace in the Valley" when he felt a connection to the world of the spirit. Neither did he lie, steal, or swear in public or in the presence of women or children, but there was something about formal religious services that kept him away. My mother never gave up, though. Each time we moved, she would say, "We should find a church and go." He agreed. But we never did.

My father had been raised by a father whose soul was seemingly filled with joy, a simple, gentle man who found the grace of God's creation in the land and the animals upon it. My paternal grandfather greeted each day gladly, his eyes constantly twinkling, his mood eternally sunny. My grandmother, conversely, was a rigid woman, perhaps so confident of right and wrong that she needed no church. From that pair, my father left home holding hard to the beliefs that the God of Moses ruled the Universe, and the Ten Commandments were law enough. Oddly, by the time he had two sons, he had seized on the idea that his children needed more religious training than he had to offer by example—some sort of wisdom he could not give but could not admit to lacking—and so he always found a way for us to attend Sunday school.

I could have said I don't want to go, when it came to those classes. But, under my father's orders, I still would have gone. In fact, though we never did, our family could have easily found a church to attend. The military bases which I had grown up on had churches, and there were chaplains plucked from every flower in God's garden ready to praise His creation. There were Roman Catholic priests and Jewish rabbis for those faiths, and for the third category, which the military then lumped together as Protestant, there was a minister who might be any breed from Baptist to Lutheran to Episcopalian.

Besides the generic Sunday school on those military bases, I had gathered up my theology from celebrating Christmas and Thanksgiving, from my mother's admonition to remember the Golden Rule, and from reading the parables of Jesus in the pages of the red-letter New Testament I had been given by an army chaplain. I loved that little red-letter version and kept it for decades, a souvenir of one of those innocuous Sunday school lessons. If Jesus said it, I thought, that was all I needed to know. Fundamentally, though, my ethics came from my father's belief that he was god in his house, one in which no lies, no theft, and no blasphemy would be tolerated.

In the green summer of 1960, in the first weeks following my return home, nearly every preacher around the Hurley community came to visit. The year before, when we first moved to the farm, our family had heard the question, "Where you all go to church?" asked repeatedly.

Those questions soon tapered off, and a measure of acceptance for our lack of religion seemed evident.

Now the invitations began again, and, looking back, I suppose each one felt I should be eager to pray at the altar, either in praise for my survival or in petition for my healing. The invitation I accepted came from a high school classmate named Tim McManus, the only child of a widow who owned a large farm. Tim could have tossed his high school diploma on the shelf and started out in a debt-free farming operation, but his ambition was to be a missionary.

Tim might not have called it "ambition." "God has called me to the mission field," is the way he and his fellow believers would have said it. During his last year in high school while I was busy flying the iron lung, Tim had joined a fundamentalist church, one which believed Protestantism didn't begin with Martin Luther but rather with Anabaptist disciples ordained by the Savior Himself. Then, after he graduated, Tim enrolled in theological school at a religious college in Springfield, Missouri.

It was becoming clear that disability was isolating, and so whatever unfathomable misgivings my father may have had toward organized religion were overshadowed by his desire to get me out of the house. At least at Tim's church I would see and interact with people, with someone other than family and an occasional visitor. As for me, still in my passive crip stage, I didn't much care one way or another, which is the wrong reason to go to church, but I liked Tim, and I appreciated his interest.

In my heart, though, I was apprehensive about launching my crippled self into a public arena. Throughout my life, I had only wanted to be the center of attention when I chose to attract notice. Now, whenever making an entrance in a wheelchair, I began to feel eyes clamped down on me from every direction, as if my green high-backed conveyance was a powerful visual magnet. I found myself surprised and nervous because of this self-consciousness, and I began to feel it was . . .

. . . *wrong, shameful, weak to ride in a wheelchair.*

God damn! Don't stare! I don't want to be in this thing. Stop looking!

Even today, I still dislike people staring. When I am in a good mood I invariably attempt to take control by greeting the person and asking a question of them. But I still believe that stares upon a visibly disabled person—a damaged creature—share the same instinct of fear and rejection and repudiation that isolates the maimed and weak from the herd.

I could not articulate that thought then. I am reluctant to believe it now.

Going to church with Tim also offered me one more tutorial not really useful in living a life disabled. I learned I didn't like to be handled by strangers, at least those of a nonmedical sort. That, of course, had nothing at all to do with religion but seems now a metaphor for the overbearing zeal with which the church's message was offered.

I was surprised at the repugnance I felt when being handled by a relative stranger, as if each touch and movement trespassed the boundaries of me. I had been lifted, tossed, and pushed by medical teams and my family for month after month. But that was in a hospital or in my home. This was in public. And it bothered me from the very first instance, even though it was for the most benign of purposes—attending church, a place where self should be subsumed into community.

Tim was a big guy, over six feet tall and more than two hundred pounds. He drove a Dodge coupe, and it was nothing for him to lift me out of my wheelchair and toss me in the front seat. At the church after he had lifted from car to wheelchair, he would motion to a couple of men, and together they would carry my wheelchair, me seated like a sultan, up the flight of stairs into the church.

I hated every minute of it, this physical reminder of my inability, my dependence, my otherness. I knew I was helpless, but I despised having it demonstrated in public. I abhorred the reminder of all I had lost.

No one built wheelchair ramps in the early 1960s. The first van I ever saw with a wheelchair lift was on the television show "Ironside," which came on air in 1967. There were no accessible bathrooms. There was only Tim and his good intentions and me—calculating my morning liquid intake so that I might make it home without having to empty my bladder, arguing internally with the unbending theology being proclaimed, and missing the voice of God.

I never met any member who wasn't at least civil, but I found the services confusing and difficult to comprehend. The words I heard preached a theology with rugged, inviolate boundaries, each tenet delivered in room-echoing volume by the pastor, a second-generation Finn from Michigan. Short and squarish, he was a Scandinavian white-blond who turned flush with passion. He was also a professor at the college's seminary, and many of his students accompanied him to Sunday worship.

The pastor and his students, good-natured and thoughtful Tim being the exception, seemed to nurture near contempt for other Protestant denominations, expressing their views with an inflexible righteousness. I disliked the fire and brimstone preaching, too much like lecturing for my tastes, and, even as unsophisticated as I was, I felt that the all-or-nothing framework expressed a spiritual rigidity unrelated to Christ's gentle words. That likable people such as Tim found passion in the restrictive religiosity of this church confused me greatly.

I stopped going with Tim after a few months. He asked why, as did some of the other young people from the church, but I couldn't tell them, not exactly. I didn't want to hurt Tim's feelings, it's true, and I disliked myself for my physical weakness and dependency. I understood I was missing my purpose, my reason, for entering God's house, but I was too naïve, confused, and self-absorbed to fathom why.

Running deeper—a paranoid, parallel undertow of feelings that I have carried with me throughout my life—was my suspicion that some people, not Tim, but some members viewed me as a project, a token of Christian charity, the little church's own private leper. And what better leper to have than one who needs saving? Or—Praise God!—even healing.

15

My parents, I think, were surprised at how few of my friends, other than Tim, visited after word got around that I had been released from the rehab center. I didn't care, at least at first. I had been in a hospital environment for almost six months, and I was anxious, even nervous, about being outside that cocoon of constant care. The re-immersion in home life, farm life, was overwhelming. I marveled at the sounds, the smells, the *ordinariness* of fresh air, sounds, movements—of dogs and cats, thunder and rain, cars and trucks rattling down the gravel road running west from Spring Creek.

And there were books to read—more Hemingway, his short stories about matadors a favorite; more Faulkner, *The Reivers* so much different from his earlier, darker work; an illustrated history of World War II; Eisenhower's *Crusade in Europe*; John Updike and John O'Hara and John Steinbeck when my mother made a trip to the library in Crane. My parents subscribed to *Life* and the *Saturday Evening Post*; my father received *Western Horseman*; the rural carrier stuck yesterday's *Springfield Daily News* in the mailbox around noon each day.

There was also a television in a setting where I could change the channel myself. Pittsburgh defeated the Yankees, Kennedy debated Nixon, and *noitartnecnoC* became *Concentration* once more. I had my own radio, one I could tune away from the farm news and country music to listen to Springfield's KICK play "Mack the Knife." Sometimes I would help my mother string beans from the garden or sit on the small porch with binoculars trained on the hills.

I wasn't surprised at the lack of visits. I knew I had no real friends, only acquaintances. I was too young to be able to articulate fully the difference between the two, but I had absorbed an instinctive comprehension of it. I had never had a lifelong friend. The constant moves making up the life of an army brat had well taught me the difference between friend and acquaintance. I related to other people only as companions in common circumstances.

Acquaintances are polite but self-interested. Friends might be boorish, ill-mannered, and demanding, but a friend is loyal and genuinely concerned.

At first, adults in the little community were regular in their visits and in their offers to help. I had always been comfortable with adults, even though children generally live at the periphery of the adult world. I'd been the overhearing type of kid, the one who hung at the edge of grown-up gatherings and listened to conversations and related to what was said, trying to learn whether it might affect or profit me.

Now I was the center of adult attention. I am certain there was an element of curiosity on their part. Fear over the disease the *foreigner*—the label most Ozark natives then had for people not born into the hills—had brought too close to their children was no longer a worry, of course. But, overriding most personal relations, there was a strong element of community in our town. People understood that a tragedy had struck our family, and they truly wanted to help. The trouble was, no matter the number of good intentions, they were no more useful than good wishes. I needed a ramp up to the porch, and my father quickly built that. There was little else that could be offered.

The days, weeks, and months passed, and I saw only two or three of my schoolmates. Granted, our farm was three miles south of town, and it wasn't as if a friend could walk a couple of blocks and knock on the door. But most of them had cars, or friends with cars, or they could have borrowed a family car. There were few that could not have visited.

When we had moved into the community the year before, I met only one person who used a wheelchair. Barbara was my age. I think she had been born with spina bifida, which left her with a significant degree of paralysis. She lived with her parents—Orie Wright, a preacher and a carpenter, and his wife, Rosie—directly across the street from the school. It was there I became acquainted with Barbara during the single semester I attended Hurley High School. Her mother pushed Barbara across the street to the campus. From there she was dependent on the students to help her up the steps to school, from class to class, and then up and down the staircase inside. It was all accomplished without direction, students converging to meet her needs of the moment.

"Where's your next class, Barbara?" someone would ask. If it was on the second level, two or three of the larger, older boys nearby would grab hold of her wheelchair and carry it upstairs, little Barbara riding like Nefertiti.

I had made it a point to be somewhere else or to hang back when it was time to assist her. Her disability made me nervous. It was as simple as that. I had never been around anyone, old or young, with a significant disability, and so I did not know how to relate to Barbara as a human being. I was too daunted by messiness, the neediness of the effort. I thought I had nothing in common with her. I could do no more than smile or nod and say "Hello."

Barbara was small and fragile, probably no more than seventy pounds, bright blue eyes shining out from a translucent face, topped by wispy curls of pale blond hair. She had grown up in a house across from the school, one more soul making up the tiny, close-knit community of Hurley. Barbara was always friendly and outgoing, recognized and accepted by everyone at school and in the town. And Barbara was not her disability. I could not see that then.

Now it was me in the wheelchair. Not yet understanding the nature of irony, I found the idea bitterly funny, with the wry emotion amplified because when acquaintances did visit, I felt left behind and thus even more isolated. It was then that I most understood how significantly our roles had changed. As much as I had felt myself, in my ignorance, different—callow Gary then would have said *better, more a whole person,* when I was around Barbara—I now assumed the role

I had assigned her: the person less-than, the one left behind. I had thought her less; now I thought myself less.

One evening a few months after I returned from Omaha, two girls with whom I had shared good-humored pranks on the school bus and in class popped in, accompanied by the younger one's boyfriend. The four of us were chatting in my living room, and one of the girls noticed a Ouija board folded up on the lower shelf of an end table.

"Let's check, Rudy," said Rita, the younger one.

"No, don't be silly," her boyfriend replied.

"C'mon. I need to know. We don't want trouble." Rita reached for the board and set it on her knees. "Put your hand on it, Rudy."

I watched from across the room. Sandy, her sister, simply shook her head.

"Ouija, will what happened in the car at the river be okay?" Rita colored as she queried the board. I could see the blush rising up her neck. "Will we be safe? Will I be safe?"

I don't know if Rudy pushed the diviner toward the "Yes" mark, but I thought the pair had gone places in the night where I had not, and now might never, venture.

Ginny, the girl I had dated shortly before my illness, did visit once. She brought her mother. And she talked about the guy she was seeing, but the words unsaid sketched out an understanding that I should take as a given, things being what they were . . .

We've all got to move on with our lives, don't we?

I had no illusions. She had visited only once or twice while I was hospitalized in Springfield, and she had never written while I was in Omaha.

During the time we were together, in those innocent nights before Vietnam, hippies, and birth control pills, Ginny wanted to please, and she was feminine enough to know she could please and do it without compromise. Each refusal came quietly. Each refusal came with a soft kiss and a look that promised more. But each refusal was absolute. Ginny was sweet fragrances in the dim light of my father's pick-up cab, eager kisses tasting of Coca-Cola, and, most of all, my hands reaching, pleading, and kneading while our tongues touched.

With others from our school and from other schools, Ginny and I often set off for the James River, or Spring Creek which fed into those hill country waters bound for the sea. There, along the banks and the gravel roads nearby, we found bonfires and rock-and-roll music from car radios tuned to stations far away. We talked, held hands, and danced, youngsters gathered there on land someone's parents owned. A mother or two sent food, and sometimes watchful fathers sat near the fire and noticed everything, noticed most of all the right moment to call out so that a couple might return hand-in-innocent-hand when summoned from the shadows.

In my living room with Ginny on that sunny afternoon, I knew whatever those nights once promised was now being submerged in the wake of Ginny's nervous chatter and her mother's silence. The older woman watched me, as if she expected me to break into tears. Ginny was still doll-like, barely five feet tall, with the same dark pixie-cut hair, a slight overbite, and brown eyes—now nervously darting about the room—which I had found so attractive. I remembered I liked it that I could reach down, put my arms under her hips, and lift her up to kiss her.

I heard Ginny's words march through her story of life going on, but I thought about love and sex, about those nights parked alone on a rural hilltop with my hands pulling her hard to me. I drifted along, thinking about the angel-soft whorls of feathery hair at her temples and at the back of her neck, and the sweet spicy smell and taste of her skin as I traced down her throat and between her heavy breasts, those breasts so precious white in my hand in the dark hours of the summer night.

I heard about the new boyfriend and his job as a lead man in the big factory in a nearby town and the new Chevy he'd bought, but, when it was my turn to talk, I began reciting stories of my adventures in the hospital, the dead and wounded, the pain, and the misery.

She had romance. I had tragedy. Together the two translated into some wry bit of human comedy.

"I'll be seeing you again," Ginny said when they left.

I did see her again. But it was eight or ten years later. She stopped by an office where I was working. She had had a miscarriage, and I think she wanted to tell me marriage wasn't quite what she thought it was going to be.

"I had another miscarriage, Gary," she said. "It looks like Susan is going to be an only child."

"I'm sorry, Ginny," I replied. "I know that's not much, is it? Just words. Words can't heal hurts."

"Mostly I just want somebody to hold me when I cry," she said.

Mostly, yes, that was it. What I wanted mostly—then, and for years before and after—was a woman to sit on my lap, put her arms around me, and believe I was the man she needed to hold her as she cried.

After Ginny and her mother left that day, my mother came from the kitchen and said, "You're making people uncomfortable, Gary. Don't tell them all those hospital horror stories that make you some sort of victim-hero. No one wants to hear that. It's too self-centered, as if you want them to pity you. You don't, do you?"

That made sense. I had grown up trying to smooth my way among adults and young people alike. I never liked to be in a situation where people were uncomfortable. Good manners had been drilled into my head. But perhaps I did want pity, not yet understanding pity wasn't going to do me a bit of good. I remember my mother's admonition left me confused.

What did people truly want from me now?

I felt as if I had become an exhibit in a freak show. I felt as if I had been chosen to play a complicated part in a community drama. People wanted to see the guy who'd crawled out of the iron lung. I could understand that. There had to be a measure of satisfaction in being able to think, Thank God, that's not my child.

And, of course, there also had to be a bit of morbid curiosity. What was it like? Were you scared? Are you ever going to walk again?

I certainly wasn't the same person these visitors knew a year before—the kid who was always ready to pull on his cowboy boots and set off on a new adventure. But I had no solid idea who the new me was—the person who had made a feverish journey through the Land of Affliction in a metal capsule.

In fact, what else did I have to share?

So there I sat, in a green vinyl and shiny chrome wheelchair, complete with a high back so that I could rest my weak neck muscles. Parked next to it, not a visitor but rather my constant companion, looking like the R2-D2 which still hid in George Lucas's imagination, stood the pneumatic belt device that drove my respiration—"Pfftt, shhhh."

Even though I then mostly believed that more than a few of my visitors were driven by curiosity, I now have grown old enough, generous enough, to grant them good intentions, to realize that despite their banal curiosity and fears and misgivings people generally tried to focus on me, expressing concern and sympathy and optimism for my recovery.

The trouble was, they were as helpless to change things as I was.

After Ginny's visit, I tried hard to follow my mother's advice. I began to deflect attention from my story, even though I still supposed it was the thing they most wanted to hear. My mother's wisdom, her insight, I now know came out of her personality, one that tried never to inflict pain and always empathized with another's discomfort. My mother also instinctively understood a truism: horror stories inspire fear and revulsion, and if you're caught up in such drama, people will pity you.

The visitors dwindled over time. People apparently lost their inquisitiveness and found the circumstances of their own lives more demanding. My world shrank as it depopulated. It became my room, the front room, and the kitchen. My escape became the television, books, and my daydreams. In good weather, my father would use the wooden ramp from the porch to move me down to the yard. Better to take a book outside when possible. In the yard, I could watch the gravel road for passers-by, nearly every one of whom waved in greeting, a country tradition. Or I could look to the east to follow the horses in the pasture. Missy, the cattle dog, would come—never wary, never curious, never voicing questions about past or future—and place her front paws in my lap so that I might rub her ears.

Those initial visits from people in the community I know now were the first lessons in the vocational course I had inadvertently signed up for—*riding lessons*, instructions for learning to live disabled after an accident or illness by being born again.

A person who arrives in this world with a disability grows aware that all that is normal for him or her encompasses them every day and every way. On the other hand, a person disabled later in life is transported—*born again*—in a territory representing another normalcy.

At age seventeen, burnt into a caricature of my former self by polio, I had been reborn a wingless phoenix. I became a crippled toddler with a new but inaccessible world to explore.

Now age eighteen and at home, I remained a child. I'd been jerked back from the freedom of manhood by disease, there to sit under the authority of my parents—my father, going about his business of providing for his wife and sons while leaving my mother to attend to my needs as she had done when I was two or three years old, right down to cleaning my bottom after a bowel movement.

Erlyne Pope Presley, wife, mother, soldiered on in love and loyalty. She escaped the pressure and the demands of my personal care rarely, seizing opportunities to work as a county election judge or as a census-taker, although even then she was bound to return home to cook for her sons and husband, a man near helpless in a kitchen. My mother seldom complained, although she would flash with frustration when my requests became demands and my indispositions deteriorated into whining. I don't remember her aging markedly, although surely she did. She had been mistaken for my sister when visiting me in the hospital and rehab center, and her younger-than-her-years appearance lasted well into her fifties.

My father farmed seven days a week, sun to sun, and Jon followed my father when he could, helping with minor chores, learning to drive a tractor or to set a milking machine onto a cow's udder. My brother looked nothing like me, grown tall and blond and square, and he fast became the son my father needed, attracting less of the paternal irritation than I had always seemed to draw upon myself, whole or damaged.

We all liked the farm less than my father did. My mother came to Missouri, I suppose, because she had promised to love, honor, and obey. But I doubt she would have chosen the isolation of country life had the decision been hers. I think she forever felt out of place, especially because we had moved into a community where a thin veneer of friendliness covered an insular society made up of twenty to thirty interrelated families. Although she'd grown up a small-town girl on the edge of the incubating Los Angeles metropolis, my mother, at least from my perspective, seemed to have "found a home in the army," as was said then. She had learned that the military was a relatively open society, with wives and families reliant upon and supportive of each other. And the official establishment itself provided the security of easily accessible resources like schools, health care, a commissary and post exchange, and recreation facilities. When we moved to the hills, my mother lost all of that, along with any chance to indulge herself with silver service from England, linens from Belgium, or the shops along the Champs-Élysées.

All my life, I knew my mother as open and guileless and loving, a woman whose heart and soul refused, at least outwardly, to dwell upon the irony that a thing she feared—poliomyelitis—had wadded up her first born child and given him back to her.

When she looked forward to her son turning eighteen and graduating from high school, she had expected to see him join the military service, or better, perhaps attend college. Instead she watched me sit in the small living room of an old rock house in an isolated county of southern Missouri, alone except for the television and books and my own fantasies, while my friends—acquaintances, really—went about becoming adults.

For them: college, jobs in factories or in construction, enlistment in the military, marriage, or work on the family farm or in town.

For me? The trappings of childhood. I was babied. Instructed. Coddled. Directed.

"I'm going to do it anyway," a typical eighteen- or nineteen-year-old male might say when his parents voiced objections. An eighteen- and then nineteen- and then twenty-year-old crip who could not crawl out of bed without assistance, a crip without friends, sat alone and futilely thought what if.

"Let's take our savings and head for California," I fantasized hearing from the lifelong friend I never had. *"I'll load you in my car. You can find someone out there to take care of you."*

Passivity might have killed me during the silent battle in my psyche for the four or five or six years I remained a newborn crip, rolling instead of toddling about in the lives of my parents.

I fought a strange, silent war—a war between me and the reality of my disability, watching as another battle raged between my parents and their future, all three of us roaming across terrain altered beyond expectation and perhaps beyond coping.

Was this struggle also one over what constituted this new family life and my place in it? If so, my mother fought quietly, without complaint, waiting on my physical needs, love in each touch, compassion in every action. My father raged silently, incoherently, fiercely resentful of what had become of his family. Jon, my brother, tiptoed around the perimeter, a child at the edge of my vision, willing to be loved and appreciated by his sibling but unable to express his desire for friendship, especially to a twisted brother too deaf to hear anything other than the silent roar of self-pity.

Alone I sat for those wasted years. Lost in self-pity, waiting for fantasies of freedom to come true, all the time ignorant of the idea that my life was mine to spend as I wished.

Alone. Wishing I could go to Vietnam. John Wayne heroic fantasies. Bullet wounds were a more satisfying adventure than polio if a young man is to ride out the remainder of his life in a wheelchair.

Alone. Night dreams of a woman. Dark eyes, black hair, ivory skin. Me—lover, passion, marriage.

Alone. Flying. High-altitude jet beneath me. Glory.

Alone. A man—seventeen, nineteen, twenty-one, twenty-three years of age—crumpled in a chrome and green wheelchair and lost in hours upon hours of a little crippled boy's flight through the dreamscapes of childhood.

16

Once a month or so during my first year home, my father would load me in the front seat of the car he had brought from Texas, a two-tone Starmist blue and Dresden blue 1957 Ford Fairlane sedan. My mother would join us, and we would drive to Springfield. There, on the ground floor of the same hospital building where I had been a reluctant passenger in the iron lung, we would meet an orthopedic surgeon who volunteered to see patients in the Crippled Children's Clinic.

The trip began with my father rolling me down the wooden ramp, the wheelchair moving backwards while he walked ahead of it, facing the opposite direction. No one since has guided my chair down a ramp in a similar fashion. He would push the wheelchair close to the car, reach under my knees and around my back, raise me up, and swing me into the front seat. My father had rarely hugged me when I was little. If I were hurt, he would steady me with a hand. If I were angry or afraid, he would challenge me with a look. Now he held me in his arms—the leftovers of what once had been a near-man almost exactly his own size—and hug me hard and close before gently lowering me into the seat.

At the clinic, we would sit and wait. Nurses and attendants would bustle through the hallways. Little children would be moved from room to room, pale and fragile, some in wheelchairs, some in a parent's arms. They were so different from me, an almost-man, painfully skinny but giving every appearance of normalcy, of being able to stand and walk. Half an hour or an hour in the waiting room, and then we would be escorted to an examination room, there to wait until the doctor would finally enter and look at what was left of me.

I always felt as if he had the demeanor of an ambulance attendant who had stumbled upon a bad wreck. I am sure he received no pay for working at the clinic, that he volunteered because of an obligation to the community and to his oath to heal the wounded. Perhaps my reaction was rooted in my own feelings of helplessness and inferiority, but I always had the impression he would rather have been in a clean, quiet operating room setting a broken bone—work that allowed him to pass along a cheerful prediction to patient and family alike that there would be a quick and complete recovery.

During one visit, I complained about my urine being pinkish, and he sent me to a urologist who told me to drink more water. At another visit, I complained of an ingrown toenail. He paused, looked at my mother, and said, "Take off his shoe and sock."

He bent down, pulled my foot into his lap, reached for a small probe, and dug out the corner of the nail. My father braced my shoulder as the pain radiated up my leg and sweat popped out on my forehead. My father's grip was his instruction to bear the pain silently.

"Hold on," my father said. The doctor continued with quick, deep thrusts of the device.

"You need to get a nail file, sterilize it with alcohol, and keep the end of these nails turned up," said the doctor, looking at my mother. Blood began to trickle down my foot, and the doctor swabbed at it.

"I'll send some of these with you." He pointed to a small box of thin wooden sticks tipped with a blob of silver nitrate. "Take one, like this," he continued. "See? Pull back here—notice the puffy flesh where it's turning purple? Burn that off." He applied the stick's end to the proud flesh at the edge of the nail, and I watched the meat wither and shrink. By then, the pain was centered in my stomach. I swallowed.

The doctor wrapped my toe, and my mother slipped on my sock. I carried my shoe. My toe throbbed so badly I couldn't tolerate the shoe's touch.

The clinic visits continued for several more months. When my nineteenth birthday arrived, it meant I was no longer a child even though I was still crippled, and we ceased to make the trips.

I didn't care. From my passive perspective, nothing much worthwhile occurred during the visits, other than the repair of the ingrown toenail. I suppose my parents were reassured because no one warned of problems looming over the horizon of permanent disability, but I also think they were confused. What I know now is that someone should have taken us into a room, closed the door, and said, "*See him in the chair? That's it. That's his life. Help him get educated for a job he can do sitting down, and then tell him to stop waiting around wasting time being a victim and start living.*"

In the meantime, there were other things to be accomplished. In August of the year I returned from Omaha, my mother had driven to the high school to find out what might be necessary for me to graduate. I had enrolled in the middle of my junior year only three credits shy of what Missouri demanded of its high school graduates, but polio had hunted me down before I completed ten weeks of my senior year.

At my mother's request, the school set up two courses to meet graduation requirements. I studied at home. I already had a copy of the yearbook from the class of 1960, what would have been my senior year. The book was dedicated to me, the missing man. But now when I finished with the two courses, my diploma would say 1961. It didn't make any difference. I had attended so many schools—thirteen that I can count over eleven years beginning with kindergarten in Japan—that I never became attached to any of my hundreds and hundreds of classmates. School was forever a matter of learning, asking questions, and bringing home report cards my parents always told me could be much better.

Now I would study alone, complete the papers and tests, and my mother would take the material to school on her trips to town. I worked at my own pace, paying so little attention that I cannot now remember the subjects I was required to study in the two courses, but apparently passed the tests without problem.

Given the culture of disability in that era, comprised of a varying mixture of pity and low expectations, I expect I would have received a high school diploma even if I had turned in blank papers. I studied in a vacuum, with no other students around and no visits from any teacher. An instructor may have called to check on me, or I may have called an instructor with a question. I doubt it. The disease—that thing called infantile paralysis—may have taken away most of my physical abilities, but my tendency to live inwardly had hardened.

The textbooks were comprehensive and easy to follow, and our family owned a new set of the *Encyclopedia Britannica*, all twenty-four volumes racked neatly in a walnut case. I might need to make a few notes on the Missouri Compromise, but I could also pause to read about heraldry, hieroglyphics, and horses.

I finished the two high school courses, and the school sent me a diploma. With it, it turned out, I became eligible for state-sponsored vocational rehabilitation services. My parents were cheered by that news. Barbara, my original classmate, may have learned about the services and told the school administration. Or the school may have reported my status to the state. All I knew was that my father said, "We'll be going to Galena tomorrow to meet with some man from the state rehabilitation agency."

I recall the traveling representative of the state agency as a square man. Don Kendrick was perhaps five feet ten inches tall and seemed more than half that wide—a box of a man—all broad shoulders, thick waist, and heavy legs. He even combed his hair in a style that made his head appear square. He gave me aptitude tests, and I answered questions. Kendrick asked what I wanted to do, and I groped for answers. I'd always wanted to be a pilot, but I had known by the time I entered my teens that my less-than-perfect eyesight would disqualify me. I simply could not conceive, given my degree of disability, that any sort of education or profession could outweigh my paralysis and allow me to make my way in the world alone.

How could I do anything worthwhile if I could do nothing for myself?

After all, I was then physically disabled to the extent that I required attendant care, and I think I subconsciously recognized that things were never going to change. The issue came up in conversation with

Kendrick during one of our first meetings, and Kendrick mentioned that a few major state universities were undertaking programs to offer accommodations for students with disabilities—accessible dormitories, ramps, elevators. He went on to say that the University of Missouri had taken notice. No one mentioned attendant care.

Who would help me in and out of bed? Who would drive me? Who would . . . ?

There were dozens of questions and only a few answers. The questions were premature at that point anyway. I was still regaining physical strength. However, the true problem wasn't my physical disabilities but rather my failure to comprehend that a crip was capable of caring for himself or arranging care for himself, of functioning as an independent human being, albeit one who would require occasional assistance.

No one told me, "There is a way for a quadriplegic to survive as an independent person."

Instead, I accepted the perfection of my dependency.

I have always hated the term *wheelchair-bound*. I hear it, and I visualize people tied in chairs, tortured, unable to flee from evils lurking about—forever tied and forever helpless. I remember Kendrick and his words about universities becoming accessible to people with disabilities, and I realize that I *used* a wheelchair, and I was *bound* by my own timidity.

When he didn't get an immediate enthusiastic reaction, Kendrick suggested that the most useful alternative in the meantime would be correspondence courses from the University of Missouri.

And that's how I began to fill my days. I studied. I studied algebra and accounting, English and American government. I chose them— or more accurately agreed to study them—because each was a prerequisite for other, higher-level courses. I chose them not realizing that they would be the only college courses I would ever take.

"What do you think you would like to do?" Kendrick had asked.

I didn't know, of course. Few twenty-year-old people are perceptive about life choices. A twenty-year-old woman might think she wants to be a wife and a mother. Let another twenty years pass, and that woman might think she made a fool's choice. Obviously, I knew I wasn't going to be a construction worker or a soldier or be involved in any other profession that required physical strength or even simple dexterity.

"I don't know," I replied. "Maybe a teacher. History teacher. I like history." That was the first job that came to mind that I imagined could be carried out sitting down.

My parents were in the room with us. No one replied. A moment passed and then Kendrick said, "Well, you'll need to get the general education courses done first."

Teacher? Yes, because teachers can sit and accomplish their work. Objectivity from the subconscious, it seems. At this point I wasn't sure what was going on with me physically—I believed, and I didn't believe, that I would be paralyzed forever—and so it wasn't a reasoned choice. No one had ever said outright, *Get used to the chair, kid. You're never going to walk again.* That might have been cruel, but it might also have been helpful.

Of course, aggressive education programs for people with disabilities and social integration would have been more useful, but this was the early 1960s. Cuba and Camelot dominated the headlines, and the nation had yet to grant full civil rights and complete access to African Americans let alone people with disabilities.

I knew I couldn't walk, at least for the foreseeable future.

Teach me shorthand and typing. A man can be a secretary or somebody's assistant.

I knew I was gaining strength slowly, nearly imperceptibly, but it had yet to sink in, to bore a hot hole through the door hiding reality, that I would ride out the remainder of my life on wheels—to measure this thing we call disability not in days or weeks but in years and decades.

Jeweler? Yeah, a watchmaker. Like the kid—what was his name?—the one who smoked so damned much at the rehab center. I could do that. Or an electronics technician, maybe.

Somewhere in the muddy riverbed of my psyche there must have lurked a creature who understood that instruction in mathematics, language, and social sciences was only a distraction. That creature waited, silent, patient, ready to help with the most important lessons—riding lessons.

. . . .

When I wasn't studying or completing a paper, I read—books, of course, and the magazines and newspapers my parents received, but I also began to subscribe to *Harper's Magazine* and the *Atlantic Monthly*. One of the university's correspondence course instructors had criticized my references to the *Saturday Evening Post* and *Reader's Digest*. I felt patronized, but I was smart enough to realize that any reference to my father's *Missouri Ruralist* or *Western Horseman* would do little to improve my grade. Outside of homework, I reread nearly all of Faulkner, fascinated by *The Sound and the Fury*, and his chronicles of the misfits of Yoknapatawpha County. I discovered John Hersey; my family had visited both Nagasaki and Hiroshima. I read Norman Mailer and James Jones, whose *From Here to Eternity* read much like my father's stories about his first enlistment. I also discovered Kurt Vonnegut and Flannery O'Connor.

For years, I kept a series of stenographer's notebooks with titles, authors, and date completed of every book. Nothing else. Three lines. A space. Three lines for the next book read. It was as if completing a book—during those years I *always* completed any book I began to read, a talisman I held onto whether the pages contained trash or treasure—meant more than experiencing the words. It was a thing accomplished by someone who seemed to accomplish little.

I typed my lessons on an old Underwood my father had bought for me, and then I often typed two or three or four more pages to help strengthen my hands and coordinate my limited arm movement. Soon, I began typing every day, lessons or not, sometimes for two or three hours straight. I typed, and I wrote, stream-of-consciousness ramblings about what was, what had been, and what never would be—page after page without knowing anything about William James and his psychological theories or James Joyce or Jack Kerouac and the Modernist movement. I wrote about politics, prayer, and the pieces of me broken apparently never to be reassembled. Hundreds and hundreds of pages over two, three, or four years until I could beat out forty or fifty words a minute using only the first three fingers on each hand.

I don't know what became of those pages. I would like to read them again. All those absent words, thoughts, feelings haunt me. Who was I then? I suspect the boxes of notes were tossed out when our family moved in 1968 to a smaller acreage at the edge of Hurley, or in 1972 when we moved to a ranch house on twenty acres adjoining an orchard east of Aurora. I know the boxes were missing in 1988 when I moved, alone, after my parents died.

No doubt the pages were juvenile scribblings, free-form words assembled into unfocused thoughts, clogged with rotten grammar and stumbling syntax. Lost now, those words, those reminders of all the things I did not recognize about my immigration into the land of disability.

Remembering this, thinking about all that my family sacrificed in service and in dreams, I think it is probably best that I do not have those typed notes from so long ago. I carry enough guilt for all the years my disability weighed down our family. I would hate to read those pages and realize that I was so caught up in confusion, self-pity, and passivity that I remained ignorant of all that I took from my mother, father, and Jon. I am shamed enough by my self-absorption during those early years. I need no written reminders.

I see all that I took. I see all that they gave. There is grief enough resting in the shadows of selfishness and selflessness.

. . . .

For years after I returned from the rehabilitation center, I lived within the confines of my family and roamed in my imagination. Occasionally, we ventured out to rodeos and horse shows, or I accompanied my parents to Springfield to shop or went along with my father as he would buy and sell livestock and equipment.

On those days, my father would lift me into the front seat of his pickup truck and we would drive from one county to another because he had heard about dairy cows, hogs, or machinery on the market. We would eventually turn into the parking lot of a livestock auction or swing down a gravel driveway and into a barn lot. If we approached a farm, there would always be a dog, but my father was never afraid. He would shut off the truck and climb out, the dog barking, circling around looking for a heel to nip, and I would watch from my perch on the front seat as the farmer came out to meet him. There would be a handshake. Perhaps my father would light a cigarette—a Winston rather than a Camel at that time in his life, the click-clank of his Zippo lighter ever-familiar—and the two would wander off to the barn or a corral.

I would be alone for fifteen minutes or half an hour, and I would descend into the part of myself that had grown stronger, deeper, a more secure refuge during my isolation, a place where fantasy offered most of the scenery.

I had always been a sly and somewhat stilted social creature—the sort covered in an exoskeleton of conviviality rather than possessing a truly empathetic heart—before polio paralyzed me. Itinerant army brats either become that sort of social pond-skater or are thorough misfits. I had the talent of acclimating myself to nearly any group, knowing nothing was permanent, knowing I only had to slip into the contemporary attitude and shuffle along with the crowd.

My parents had experienced stable childhoods, at least through their school years—one house, one school, one town. They could recall classmates, teachers, and neighbors. During the early days of my paralysis, I began to compare their upbringing to mine and thought perhaps my travel-filled childhood made it easier for me to tolerate the isolation that came in a package with polio.

The question that lives on these decades later, reaching out from self-absorption, is if my parents' memories of their childhoods made it more difficult for them to accept that disability had turned me into a hermit. Did they regret the choices—the career in the army, the life on the farm—that left me with little chance to develop intimate friendships?

Actually, at that point, I found the isolation validating in some respects, a fact I never shared with my parents. Both would have seen it as another facet on the diamond of self-pity. I took a weird pride in my predicament. I found comfort in contriving a fantasy that my simple existence proved I had mined a heroic quality from within; I fancied I had survived through an act of will, an act of bravery.

That contradictory delusion—heroic, even though dependent—overlooked the fact that I would wither and die in bed—or wheelchair-bound—if I did not have someone to watch over me.

Helpless babies are not heroic.

These fantasies kept me from recognizing that my parents were the true champions—the two who had the heart to sacrifice a significant part of their lives to assure mine, nurturing me without complaint. Perhaps it would have done no good to speak of that which was missing, then or later. Mine was simply the same undeniable choice faced by all the hard-worn country folk and hill people whose blood ran in our veins. Get up, grab your bootstraps, and set out to do what must be done.

. . . .

More than that one conversation, that one confrontation of all we had lost as a family, was missing.

I had seized upon the idea that the absent thing was that which had been destroyed by the polio—an element of my physical self—and that it had handicapped my parents' lives. By turns confused, frustrated, and guilt-ridden, I pulled further within myself, sustained by my delusions and daydreams, refusing to confront the fact that remaking my life might require others to give up even more of their own dreams so that I might act in my selfish interests.

And there was one more question no one voiced. *Was I worth it?*

I doubt there is a person alive who, in the terrain I was then exploring, would not hear the same subconscious whispers . . . *better off dead.*

Of course, during my first postparalysis years, I tended to phrase it in a fashion resonating with self-pity—*I wish I had died!*

The dynamic of that thought is revealing and ugly. If I truly believed it, I could have killed myself, but I didn't make that choice, preferring passivity to action, no matter how wrong. In fact, even as I expressed the idea silently to myself, I slowly began to comprehend it was simply another of those self-absorbed reactions to circumstances I lacked the will to change. After all, there were firearms in the house, albeit in my parents' bedroom. There were flammable fluids. There were razors. There were pills.

I might have stared at the abyss from the rim of the iron lung, but I was afraid to die. Many of us are, but my fear had an ugly twin—I was also afraid to live as fully as possible.

Even hamstrung by poverty—at this point in my recovery, I had no money except that given to me—I could have telephoned my grandparents, an aunt, or one of my cousins. I could have asked, begged, one of them to help me move to California or Oklahoma and give me a place to stay. Realistically, though, my options were restricted to suicide or the status quo—living as a dependent child in my parents' home. No one would challenge my father's rejection of any initiative on my part to leave, to be on my own. And rightfully so. Even if I had demanded to be driven to Springfield, dumped at a hospital, and turned over to whatever authorities who would have had me, my parents would have refused.

My father resented the idea that I could not develop a plan for my future—that I was willing to sit, eat food prepared by my mother, and wait for them to lift me from bed to chair, dress me, and then reverse the process twelve hours later—but at the same time he was pessimistic about my prospects.

About the time I finished ten or fifteen college correspondence credit hours, Kendrick, the vocational services counselor, again brought up the subject of enrolling at one of the universities offering accommodations for students with disabilities. I know now there was an opportunity. I regret that I lacked the will to take it.

That second conversation with Kendrick occurred a year or more after we first met, and I cannot remember that he mentioned the availability of personal attendant care at that time. All my parents and I understood is that I certainly couldn't survive independently. In a practical sense, if I had had access to a power wheelchair and lived on campus, I might have gotten by with two hours of help in the morning and an hour of assistance at night, but our family couldn't afford to hire someone to provide those services.

I believe my father would have considered it, if we had possessed the financial resources. My father's family, like my mother's, had scraped by during the Depression, watching as the Dust Bowl blew away the last remnants of prosperity, and the bankruptcies and bank collapses left him appreciative of how greatly money affected survival. And we were all still early in our understanding that permanent disability is best combated by money, and lots of it. My father, though, was thoroughly self-reliant. He clung to the idea that he alone—meaning with the help of my mother, of course—had the responsibility to provide for my care. We were not welfare cases.

That confused me. I had no conception of how to be self-reliant, even though he had raised me without allowing me to use the word "can't." Since I had been paralyzed before I grew old enough to leave home and live on my own, I had never accomplished all the mundane transactions of daily life—renting an apartment, finding a bank, signing up for utilities—that young people do in the natural order of things. Now my father preached determination and discipline in the face of my descent into dependency, but his automatic response to any suggestion of me living independently was negative.

Perhaps his idea, and maybe my mother's too, was that physical self-sufficiency is the foundation of independent living—that a person has no right to ask another person for help with the daily necessities.

Upon hearing Kendrick's plan, could my parents have sold the farm and moved our family to a town near a university?

Obviously so, but I didn't ask my father to do so. I had no right. I might dream of freedom, but I never felt he should be obligated to sacrifice his happiness, his life, to pursue the possibility that I might someday accumulate the skills necessary to support myself as a person with a disability.

Could my mother have moved with me to a town with an accessible university, there to be my caretaker?

She could have taken a part-time job so that we might afford an apartment and other essentials. I could have earned a degree in four or five years. We could have spent holidays and the summers at home. I didn't ask that—a request that would have forced her to choose between one son or her husband and another son. Nor did she offer.

If the fracture of the family for my sake was discussed in the black hours of the night as my mother and father lay together in their marriage bed, I never knew it.

All I felt during that period was constant frustration, overwhelming guilt, unavoidable responsibility—all surrounded, pushed, driven by an unfocused desire to do something, anything.

Part of me wanted to seize the opportunity, to push myself past what I conceived of then as my physical limits, to demand of my parents a sacrifice I had no right to ask. Another part of me wanted to shout, "Don't do it for me. Not for me. I don't deserve it. I'm sorry I've screwed everything up, but I don't know how to make it any better. Tell me! I'll do it. I promise."

Part of me was afraid—afraid to leave the care of people who loved me and put myself at the mercy of people I did not know, people desperate for a few dollars that could be earned lifting, bathing, and dressing me.

In my confusion, I kept silent. In my passivity, I allowed the decision to be made for me by not deciding for myself. I was doubly paralyzed, circumscribed in my outlook, unable to look past what was, unable to see what could be. I could have leaped at—demanded—the chance to attend a university. I doubt it would have broken my parents' marriage, but I know it would have aggravated the emotional turmoil of a family learning to live with loss.

I found it odd that it was my mother who worried most about my missed opportunity to take one step toward independence, to salvage something from the debris of my life. It had been my mother who had babied me as I fought to cope with disability, while my father had pushed and prodded when I expected to be waited upon or otherwise acted the victim. She had tolerated complaints. He had demanded strength. Now, at this glimmer of opportunity, there was a mordant twist of perspective. My mother pushed for a solution to be found. She believed that I could accomplish more than my damaged body might indicate. It was my father who seemed to withdraw into pessimism, perhaps believing that I could not function outside the arms of the family.

I acquiesced to his pessimism.

I have no one to blame but myself. I was paralyzed, but I forgot I might summon up the strength to choose independence.

I know my parents were dealing with a situation so foreign as to be incomprehensible. Both came from environments in which a person with a disability was "a shut-in" or "an invalid"—environments where there might be a family friend with an aunt who never was "quite right," an aunt who now lived with a grandmother and helped string beans or shuck corn.

In fact, though, society as a whole continued to cling to a circumscribed perspective of disability. Only a few universities saw the future.

I know my parents believed I was more than a shut-in. I was also less, given the intractable nature of my physical dependency. But I was their son, and blood has obligations all its own, and they tried their best to live up to them.

And so I didn't go to a university, and I lived to tell about it, living in solitude, recuperating physically and struggling emotionally, living through days, weeks, months, years within myself, living closed off to the idea that commitment and sacrifice might be possible on my part as well as my parents', living closed off to the understanding that my parents could not care for me forever, that they might not outlive me, that an education would be the first step toward sustaining myself.

None of that occurred to me. After all, I was a crip.

Crips die early.

17

When the issue of my leaving the farm to attend college was decided by not deciding, Kendrick, the vocational rehabilitation counselor, kept whatever opinion he had of my cowardice and my parents' conservatism to himself. If he thought it a good opportunity missed, he didn't turn his back on me. He soon found another enterprise that finally launched me out of the house, one he felt so promising that he took time to drive out to our farm.

"Here's the thing," Kendrick said, sitting on the red sectional couch my mother had moved from house to house during my itinerant childhood. He leaned forward and crushed out one of the multiple cigarettes he smoked during our interviews. "The 3M Company wants to move into small towns with retail outlets for some of their products meant for small offices. They've got company representatives working here in Missouri. The idea is to provide training and material for handicapped people to market their stuff."

I remember the name of the program as something like Community Business Associates. The idea was to put photocopy machines in the hands of people with disabilities, persuade a local business to offer free office space on a temporary basis, and turn disability into a community resource. This was 1965 or 1966, and the 3M copier to be distributed for use in the program was called the Thermofax. It relied on special imaging paper but, using a special film, the little machine could reproduce transparencies as well as photocopies. Normally, the transparencies were meant for overhead projectors, but some enterprising MBA at 3M corporate headquarters had dreamed up the idea of inserting them into light boxes. Each CBA operator would have a number of boxes to rent out as lighted displays in all their eight-by-ten glory. The rental fees would be supplemented by selling personalized transparencies—which meant a Community Business Associate would be able to offer both product and service.

With the photocopy machine, a half dozen light boxes, access to a telephone, and a minimal investment in random office supplies if there was other money to be invested, a person with a disability could be turned loose to mine community goodwill for an income, to be generated at fifteen cents a copy. That was the loss leader. The real money was to be generated by renting the light boxes and printing new advertising inserts on a regular schedule.

The 3M corporation's representative for Missouri was named Jim, a man about thirty, with stylishly trimmed blond hair. Whenever we met, he was dressed in an executive-in-training dark suit. He quickly signed me up for the program—no aptitude test necessary. That was an error on everyone's part. The assumption was that my fanny in a wheelchair was qualification enough, and a detailed loose-leaf training manual I received was meant to jump-start my venture into the world of commerce.

Jim worked hard among store owners and other business people, country folk who wore gabardine slacks and open-collared shirts to work every day, and he soon found me space in a one-man insurance office in the town of Crane, about ten miles east of our farm. The agreement was that I would answer the agent's telephone and take messages; in return I would be allowed to use the telephone and set up a display of office supplies and install a table and shelf for 3M's photocopy machine.

I commuted to work through the good offices of my parents, three miles up Highway CC, a gravel road soon to be paved, and then nine more miles west and south from Hurley to Crane, once a prosperous Missouri-Pacific Railroad town. My father would finish the morning milking, by which time my mother would have me out of bed and dressed, and then he would lift me into the front seat of the car or up into the cab of his pickup and drive me to the little red-brick office and unload me.

Later, he found a used Chevrolet Corvair van, and my mother was able to ramp the wheelchair into the space where the van's middle seat had been removed. My father traded a white Mercury coupe for the van, and it was the only occasion during Jon's life that I remember my brother displaying any irritation that my disability took precedence. He was rapidly approaching the age to obtain his own driver's license, and he complained voraciously to my mother that he wouldn't—couldn't—drive the boxy Corvair van on dates or to social events. My father understood. When Jon was old enough for a license, my father bought him his own pickup.

I seldom missed work. Whatever damage poliomyelitis had done, I remained generally healthy. I had a rare cold, or perhaps the flu, but I never had any of the kidney problems or pressure sores common to a quadriplegic who regularly spent fourteen hours a day in a wheel-chair. As for getting to work after a snow storm or other bad weather, my father was the sort who rarely feared bad driving conditions. Too much snow? A low-water bridge washed out after a downpour? Dad would load me into his pickup instead of the van, and we'd set off to follow what we called "the back way"—an adventure composed of narrow gravel roads, tire chains, and my father's refusal to be intimi-dated while behind the wheel.

Once at the office—a Victorian-era storefront with high ceilings decorated with engraved tin panels—I would be on my own until late in the afternoon.

I hated it. And I loved it.

I loved it because once again, after years of isolation, I was among people. Strangers, in fact, people I had never seen, people who didn't know me or my history. I had a chance to listen. Country people nearly always have something to say about the weather, about crops, about the history of the land and the people.

I listened because I had grown up listening, both in my family and in the society of army families. But, in my wheelchair, unable to stand, shake hands, and say, "Been good to see you. Got to be on my way," I also found myself to be a trapped audience. I soon became a willing and attentive one, happily immersed in the culture of small town politics and personal problems. It seemed as if Edgar Lee Masters's *Spoon River Anthology* had come alive.

I loved the tall tales and the gossip, but I hated the idea of what I was supposed to be accomplishing. I understood the concept—that a thing called Community Business Associates might allow a person with a disability to become independent—and I know it may have been a worthwhile concept. I also know I was the wrong person then to implement it. I didn't believe in myself, or my skills, or the opportunity. Instead, I believed success meant I had to rely on the disguised charity of one business owner or another—that I was a project. Each time I tried to convince someone that a small light box might boost sales, each time I cajoled a few dollars from one merchant or another, I was haunted by the idea that the enterprise was entirely make-work.

What was the logic behind 3M's development of the idea? Why did the huge corporation set out to prove that an insignificant niche business would be appropriate for a person with a disability? I think the idea might have worked for someone more attuned than me to the process of buying and selling. Businesses spring up and grow where nothing has flourished before, and it takes a person—and disability has nothing to do with this—with vision to see new opportunities.

What wasn't explored in the CBA concept, at least in my case, was the idea that a person with a physical disability gains ground in other areas of life—that is, becomes better at those things unaffected by his disability. In my case, I could still dial a telephone and make calls, but I was no businessman, and I certainly was no salesman. Sales—advertising yourself, your service, and pushing a product no matter how peripheral it might be—was the dynamic behind the 3M idea.

But neglecting CBA sales calls and interacting with people who came into the insurance agency gave me time to take an interest in the business going on around me. I soon found myself doing more for the agent than taking messages. I began filling out routine forms and doing his filing, enough so that he handed me a set of manuals and said, "Study these, get familiar with the forms and process, and I'll let you do more for me part-time. We'll work out some sort of wage when you're ready."

I was ready that day, but the wage I would eventually earn, written up as contract labor, amounted to less than the minimum wage of the era. I didn't care. I didn't have to sell anyone anything. All I needed to do was answer the telephone, fill out an automobile coverage transfer form occasionally, complete a claim form sometimes, and make notes about the more complex problems to give to the guy who was to become my first boss.

The agent's name was Harold Connolly, and he was new to the game. He had returned to the little rural town where he had grown up from the big city of Houston, Texas, where he had been in the money as a broker for a prosperous wholesale company. His father had died, and his mother had asked him to take over the family insurance agency. The only thing left of the old man was his surname in blue paint on the plate glass window, his widow's questions about the state of the business, and a restored antique muzzle-loader hanging over the front door.

Harold was tall, well over six feet, with wavy receding hair, a constant smile, and a wife who appeared unhappy about being exiled to a small midwestern town. I felt happy—useful—working for Harold.

A year passed, and I neglected the 3M business more each day, making only the occasional photocopy or selling a few reams of bond paper. Jim, the corporation's representative, would stop by every six months and chide me for my lack of interest by reciting CBA success stories in other communities. A year or two after I had set up shop he told me he was being transferred to another corporate division, and someone new would be assigned to my account. I never heard from anyone at 3M again. I cannot remember what happened to the photocopier, although I continued using it for years, putting a small sign in the insurance agency's window that said "Photocopies 15¢."

I know I disappointed Jim, and perhaps some forward-thinking executive in 3M, but through their efforts I did find a place in the world, a place where on-the-job training and independent study helped me qualify for a state license as an insurance agent. I never owned an agency, but I began to earn a decent wage. I was a clerk, a paper-pusher, but a good one. The old brick building on a side street in a little town, once a vital link in the prosperous Missouri-Pacific Railroad line, had opened a door to a young man in a wheelchair and showed him a job he could do.

It wasn't much in the scheme of things, but at least in a small way, at least for eight hours a day, I was taking care of people's needs instead of relying on them to take care of mine. I know that now. I wish it hadn't taken me so long to recognize it.

Small-town America was another country then, post-Eisenhower and pre-Reagan, before church folk could watch porn on late-night cable television, before a farm boy with a mouthful of Skoal played gangsta rap on the stereo in his pickup truck, before grandmothers had e-mail. The only clouds on the horizon that hinted at storms of immense social proportions were the draftees returning home from Vietnam with ribbons and wounds. Only the banker wore a tie to work; lawyers wrote wills and settled probate cases instead of defending meth cooks; and the town marshal was an old man with a bad hip. When it was time for merchants to cope with itinerant beggars and troublemakers, they relied on their own wits and maybe the muscles of clerks and customers.

Among the traveling con artists, there was one lonely grifter who intrigued me, whose regular visits to the country town made me think about the nature of work and charity, about the difference between reality and appearance.

The man visited Crane every two or three months to harvest a money crop. When he first appeared at our office—or, at least the first time I met him—he walked in wearing a narrow-brimmed fedora-style hat atop a tidy white short-sleeve dress shirt, tie, and gabardine slacks. When I noticed him later that winter, he sported a trench coat. His colors were muted tans and grays, and the expression on his round, clean-shaved face was always neutral.

"Help Support A Deaf Person." That was his business card, light gray, heavy dark embossed print. No name. No office telephone or address. The reverse side displayed illustrations of the hand signs for the letters of the alphabet.

"Hello, may I help you?" I asked the first time he came into Harold's office.

He stopped in the middle of offering his card as I pushed back from my desk and exposed my legs and my wheelchair. Then he looked around, paused but finally gave me his card so that I might read it. I noticed he was carrying a small container with packets of pencils stapled to a small section of white cardboard.

"What can I do for you, sir?" I asked, looking at him directly.

He paused, pointed to my wheelchair, and then to his ears, finally raising his hand and shaking one finger side to side in a negative motion. Then he turned and left.

"You should've yelled something crazy when his back was turned," my boss said. Harold had stopped by at noon to watch the office while I ate a sandwich. "He's been coming around for years. Sometimes I take a package of pencils and give him a couple of bucks, but I bet he's got a new car hidden on some side street waiting to take him to the next town."

"Why do you say that?"

"Think about it," Harold replied. "Four or five little towns a day. Twenty bucks a town. That's two thousand a month tax-free. Not a bad racket. Hell, I bet he can even hear."

The deaf man never returned, not even when other people were in the office whom he might tap. I would see him occasionally navigating the streets. Once he glanced in the window as he was moving down the sidewalk, and I waved for him to come inside. He didn't.

I would have liked to grab some scratch paper and write down a few questions for him.

"Why do you do what you do?" I suppose that would have been the first one. I would have had a dozen other questions, had he been willing to write down the answers, but each of them would have been a single query wearing many masks.

"Don't you feel this is a little too close to begging?"

It was during that period that I first began to understand that salesmanship, regardless of the help offered by the 3M Corporation, wasn't part of my nature. I could never separate a legitimate purchase from an act of altruism. Was my business service—were its customers—the equivalent of Deaf Man's enterprise?

Sometimes, jealous of his mobility, I lapsed into envious resentment and labeled him Deceit Man—either a liar or a lazy man, taking the easy way out, relying on disguised charity rather than doing something useful like digging ditches or working as a carpenter or a welder or even an accountant. A person doesn't need to hear to add and subtract.

Conversely, I sometimes thought that what he chose to do served some purpose. When Deaf Man met the generous at heart or the gullible, he became a vessel through which those people might create good energy by reaching out in compassion. On the other hand, when he confronted the cynical, the angry, and the disbelieving, he offered them another brick to add to the wall that defended their truths.

Deaf Man didn't want my money, but I began to think I owed him thanks. He walked through that office door at a time in my life when I was beginning to measure the extent of my usefulness in the world. I was stunned that he would equate my position with his own—that I too existed as an object of charity. His quick comparison had forced me to examine the nature of the self-esteem I had constructed to hide my disability, esteem earned by working as a low-paying clerk.

I had yet to learn that I had been drafted into an army that throughout most of human history had sustained itself by begging. I did not comprehend that feelings of self-worth and accomplishment must be generated from within one's own spirit, that I had to construct my own identity and then defend it, that I would ever be challenged to prove it was real and valuable.

Gifts carry obligations, both to giver and recipient. Throughout my life, I had chosen only the obligations I felt strong enough to meet. I didn't go looking for challenges, especially the sort that required me to give of myself. That trait sometimes also made it difficult for me to see where charity was necessary. I justified that by believing I was reluctant—that I rarely offered assistance because I didn't demand it from other people.

Until the wheelchair.

Until I became an unwanted rolling responsibility.

I had always hated charity, but I'd begun to seem to need it.

Or at least its cousin—generosity of spirit.

There I sat, looking to all the world—even to those on the receiving end of society's benevolence—as if I were a suitable target for sweet largess. I didn't want it. I couldn't accept it.

I understood then, and still believe now, that it takes a certain grace to accept charity, a grace I could not find within me during that period, whether I had a cup full of pencils to sell or 3M light boxes meant to glow invitingly with one blandishment or another.

18

Somewhere between ten and fifteen years after beginning this life-long journey on wheels, I became clinically depressed. I know that now. I didn't know it then.

I only knew I could manage just enough energy to continue working, but I doubt I was a useful employee. Office hours over, I left the insurance agency, went home, sat alone in a darkened room, and looked at nothing. I did not read. I did not listen to music, leaving the Beatles, Rod Stewart, and Bob Dylan, my favorite, behind. I sat, letting the bleakness that I camouflaged in the presence of friends and strangers blank out the light. I sat until bedtime, and then I allowed myself to be tossed into bed, where I stared at nothing, blank, until sleep descended.

No one knew where to find the rope that might rescue me as I drifted down into depression's silent black hole. Talking at me didn't help. It is useless to talk to someone who either isn't listening or who doesn't care to respond.

Visitors. Interaction with family. Words rattled about the room, bouncing off my head, hours of them, days of them, but the ones I remember best were the most straightforward. "C'mon, you've got to pull yourself together!" Friends and family can say that a thousand times, or you can pay to hear it from a psychiatrist, psychologist, or minister. It's still empty talk if you decide not to listen.

"Get him a bottle of wine," my father told my mother. "Tell him to drink a glass before he goes to bed. That should make him sleepy. And that's what he needs. A good night's sleep instead of brooding all night like he broods all day."

Neither of them had any experience with clinical depression. Neither of them had ever sought counseling. Life is difficult and painful sometimes. So what?

If I hadn't been so damned depressed, I would have been surprised at my father's suggestion. My father disliked drunks. He drank, but I never noticed him intoxicated, much less liberated by the genie others found in a bottle of spirits. My father spent twenty-three years in the army, and the army runs on paper, field rations, and ammunition, but its bearings are lubricated by beer. That was his choice of alcoholic drink, especially when a day's farm work had been miserably hot. But the icy beer came only after the work was done. Overindulgence in alcohol, like overindulgence in food, was evidence of sloppy weakness, a character flaw.

I was also astonished because there was a person with a disability in our area who might have been an alcoholic. I don't know how George Williamson found himself using a wheelchair, but he had survived—perhaps even prospered—without becoming a shut-in or an invalid, terms common in that place and time. He was "crippled up," as country folk might say, the sort of man who couldn't put in a hard day's physical work but was still able to earn his keep, an admirable condition according to hill-country ethos.

Williamson had been an elected county official for decades. From the Civil War through the Great Society, any candidate chosen by the local county political committee had a job for life as long as the happy office-holder supported the party in that one-party county. In that area—actually, across almost all southwest Missouri during that period—Republicans were as much yellow dogs as any Dixiecrat you could name.

Once elected, Williamson only had to support party decisions, contribute to election funds, and keep a believable set of books for the state auditor. With that, he had a secure niche in the bureaucracy conducting the affairs of eight thousand people, assuring him an income courtesy of his friends who didn't believe in welfare but knew a man needed to put beans on the table.

I sometimes speculate, with no evidence, that he was the sort who stayed constantly under the influence of alcohol and yet functioned well enough in daily life. Even if that was somewhere in the neighborhood of the truth, I think people would have been willing to excuse his self-medication with alcohol because he was a cripple. Those sort of assumptions are often wrong, certainly. If he had an unquenchable craving for alcohol, it may have been unrelated to his disability.

I remember he could drive a vehicle, something I could not do. He could stand and walk a few steps, something I could not do either, but he relied mostly on a wheelchair. He was a small man, visibly malformed, his right leg canted outward at the knee, his spine curved forward immediately above the hips, and his weight too heavy. I remember dark, slicked-back hair, the half plastic, half metal-rimmed glasses popular in the 1950s, and a flushed complexion. If he drank more than he should, maybe the liquor was a painkiller, or maybe booze assuaged frustration, or maybe he simply liked the taste and the effect. No one cared. Williamson held office, I think, until he died or retired, and the work got done one way or another.

My father never said as much, but I sensed that on the topic of Williamson he voted with the majority—if Williamson did drink, it was to kill the pain and the frustration of a severe disability. Perhaps that's why my father believed alcohol might provide me relief, might be a substitute for the strength of will I seemed not to have.

Looking back—filtering perceptions through experience—I find it ironic that I had trouble then saying the word. To me, it was whine. Considering that I was still wrestling with self-pity, I suspect Dr. Freud might have had something to say about my ineptitude.

"Gary," my mother would say, "listen to me as I say it. It's Y-ine."

I drank a lot of wine—mostly sweet port, sometimes a dry, sharp German wine. But I never drank enough to grow drunk or enough to relieve the depression. Why was I depressed? Had the reality of my paralysis at last reached beyond the last of my conscious mental barriers? Did an inconceivable authenticity of paralysis and pain, a destroyer of hard-held delusions, finally sink to the seabed of my subconscious? I think so now. I think my inability to persuade myself that there were choices to be made, in action and in attitude, that I was free—and wholly me—in spite of paralysis may have boiled into an incessant sense of frustration and anger, and then turned into chronic depression.

For months—a year? two?—I went to work, sat quietly in the torrent of talk about rates and claims, and then returned home to brood another night away. I stopped reading. I cared nothing for television or music. I withdrew into my room and thought about killing myself. Nights. And days. I even said the words aloud in the empty room, trying to make them into an acceptable solution, but every night I would take the last sip of wine, carry the glass to the kitchen sink, and turn away to face one more night of darkness rather than an eternity of the unknown. Whether I was saved by apathy or by fear, I do not know.

If I then had seized on the idea that I was a pitiful, broken prisoner in a wheelchair, I had ignored the idea that most prisoners would willingly eat rats and bugs to stay alive. Hypnotized by despair, paralyzed by self-pity, I abdicated control of all that was left of me to the same hidden energy that powers the gazelle's kicks even as the lion drags it to earth. Life does not give up easily.

I never became an alcoholic. I never *needed* another glass. Instead, I related my predicament to the psychological aftereffects of polio, understanding that the toughest thing to chew, the hardest thing to swallow after my disability had been the loss of autonomy. That had not changed. That justified the soft, warm release of tension found in a glass of wine. But I still felt every day—every hour!—overwhelmingly frustrated and beaten down by my lack of control. I knew there was more to be lost, more of me to wash away, in those smooth bottles. I drank a glass, sometimes two, and for a few minutes before I fell asleep, the overbearing sense of despair and hopelessness became less important. One glass, or two. Somehow, by God's grace, I knew the third glass, or the fourth, or the bottle might wash away the last illusions of the minimal control I retained over my life.

I cannot recall how long depression lasted. Depressed people don't count days. I remember the two-story Victorian-era house at the edge of Hurley—the Steele place, its grounds ripe with coffee cans stuffed with greenbacks according to legend—where we lived when the darkness fell on me. We had moved to the Steele place in 1968, and we lived there until 1972.

Nor can I recall why I finally gave in and sought help from a physician. I cannot remember if I subconsciously ceded control to my parents. Did they demand that I see a doctor? Perhaps I went to a physician for another reason, and he glimpsed something in my eyes or in my demeanor. I doubt that. We lived then in a place and a time where people in need of psychiatric care were sent to the state hospital—and that only after they became catatonic or whispered paranoid delusions into the ears of their frightened family members.

I remember nothing about the why or the when. I remember only the pills that the doctor gave me to substitute for the wine.

Red pills, the size of a warped shotgun pellet. Red pills, to be shuffled from bottle to mouth and thus mark a day in another series of lost months. I suppose the pills were some early form of a monoamine oxidase inhibitor or imipramine, common then in the treatment of depression.

Cures can be worse than the disease.

Half a pill or a whole one, I held the red power on my tongue and swallowed, and then I became a zombie.

"The pills . . . the red ones you prescribed . . . make me feel . . . weird. Sluggish," I told the doctor. "Like I'm full of water, no, wet concrete. It's hard to . . . think."

"Give them time," he replied. "Your body will accommodate itself."

I spoke, and the words came from another mouth. I moved, and I felt engulfed in inertia. A sip of tea, pill swallowed, dissolving, and then release—and all the paralysis burnt into my spinal cord flooded my psyche. Depressed, I had worked. Under the influence of the red pills, I sat in the office each day. I watched myself respond in monosyllables to requests, to problems, to demands. I worked, I know, a series of Mondays through Fridays, time measured but unaccounted for, in the haze of lost weeks.

Another check-up, another complaint. The doctor offered another kind of pill. The right thing to do would have been to ask for a referral to a psychiatrist, but people deep into depression rarely make correct choices.

And so it went, support and sympathy from my mother, confusion and suppressed frustration from my father. My brother, Jon, finishing high school and moving off to college, might have been baffled, but he was too unworldly—and too busy swimming through his youth into manhood—to comprehend my predicament. I had no close friends, at least none close enough to care, and my boss needed only assurances that I would show up the next morning and sit behind my desk, there to write down legible and halfway comprehensible messages when the telephone rang.

Finally, a day came when I ignored the doctor and didn't take the little red pill. I noticed no difference, except that I felt lighter, freer, more aware of the world. Two or three days later when I felt the drowning oppression flooding over me once more, I took one. Then I skipped two more days. Or five. Then I took another, on the sixth or seventh day, when the despair and the hopelessness seemed to outweigh the prospect of the lethargy and helplessness. And then I stopped altogether.

Perhaps I had simply bored myself with anxiety and alienation. Perhaps I grew tired of depression and self-pity or, even more, of being doped into isolation.

By odd circumstance, I had stopped altogether only a day or two after I refilled a prescription for the little red pills. I counted a few more than twenty in the bottle that evening. Blood-red, mood-suppressing spheres. Twenty tiny worlds where existence might stumble forward in a stupor. Twenty chances to reduce reality to a deadly hum, all captured in a bottle I could keep in the right front pocket of my trousers.

I carried that same bottle for years, checking it occasionally, relying on its promise of utter isolation, its assurance of emotional extinction if . . . if *what*? If I lost control perhaps, or more accurately, the illusion of control.

A talisman. Twenty promises that I could escape being me and become a thing that could not act or feel and did not care.

I don't remember when I misplaced the bottle which contained those promises. Nor do I remember when I stopped feeling depressed every day.

. . . .

Chronic depression sometimes leads to suicide, and sometimes people are suicidal without being depressed. I had thought about suicide regularly for years, beginning when my comprehension of my predicament emerged in the wake of polio and pneumonia's fevers. Suicide in an iron lung would have been a slow process, I suppose, the one weapon being the refusal to eat. It would have been an ugly thing, prolonged and aggravated by forced feeding. Even as I grew in strength and began to seize upon those pleasures becoming available as I rolled about the world, I still carried the suicide demon along for the ride. As I thought about ending my life, I could not recall hearing about anyone during my childhood who had committed suicide, although there were once whispers about an army officer at Fort Bliss who was killed while cleaning his automatic pistol.

Then, a year or two after the heaviest depression began to fade from my life, I heard the story of a cruising buddy from high school. One night he drove to his ex-wife's house, parked behind her boyfriend's car, and stuck a pistol under his chin. I remember thinking, *Damn, he shot himself over a woman.*

Even though his death didn't seem worth it, didn't seem cause enough, it didn't pull me away from the selfish idea that I had better reason.

By the time I was past forty or more, having survived that extended episode of depression, I thought I knew all about despair. I was a crip, of course. And, truth told, I had yet to come to grips with the idea that my work made a difference in the world. In fact, I felt trapped by some of the less attractive dynamics of the insurance business—the cynicism, the caution, the closed-off nature demanded of me when I interacted with some customers. I felt trapped by lies, suspicion, and disrespect, and trapped most of all by anger at myself for choosing an easy job that paid good money rather than taking a chance on a challenge. A day did not pass when I did not suspect I was being lied to or when I felt people judged what I did with contempt, viewing me as the front man in a legalized scam. It is an ugly thing to live within the ebb and flow of ill will.

But as an insurance peddler, you turn skeptical if you're smart. Skeptical, yes, and—holding on hard to keep from falling into an attitude of callous cynicism—analytical about every word voiced by a customer. People generally despise the insurance industry. The more dispassionate and sophisticated can recognize that the industry is comprised of a group of cold corporations focused on the disinterested analysis of the best path to profit over loss. Those people can accept it as a business necessary in a free market economy.

On the other hand, a productive insurance agent understands that fear and misfortune are raw material, and that agent learns to look past the natural repugnance people feel when they're forced to deal, out of fear and caution, with all that is represented by the agent's product.

People are reluctant to buy insurance because they do not want to use insurance. Using insurance means that a person has encountered serious trouble, and the benefits paid by insurance can never compensate anyone fully for a loss. The situation becomes further confused when the prospective buyer learns that the best rates are reserved for those with the best claims history.

No, I never had an accident. Not in my whole life.

Through the decades I worked in insurance offices, I hated the idea that the natural course of things left me being lied to on a regular basis, left me always suspicious of people's motives. Too many people thought an accident was an accident, that there was never any fault to be assigned, especially if it was past history. People "didn't think" hitting a telephone pole was an accident. People "forgot" that they had paid a $75 fine for speeding. In spite of my ever-increasing cynicism, I never responded to lies with lies about insurance or its purpose. I didn't care enough. Let the customers attempt to disguise the fact their record wasn't accident-free or evade questions about violations. I expected it. But I never promised what I—what the company—could not deliver.

That's why it's a bitter irony that the one customer who left my office and went home to shoot herself made the choice because we both replied with the hard truth to every question we asked each other.

The woman bustled into the office late one Friday afternoon. No doubt the last hour of the last day of the normal work week is the worst time to attempt to accomplish anything in corporate America, but I was in no special hurry that fall evening. I ran down the usual questions. When I came to the one about license suspensions, she replied, "Yeah, that's a problem. I've had my license pulled for drunk driving. I need to make a filing to get it back."

That kind of story wasn't new, and I had learned not to be judgmental. In fact, I appreciated her forthrightness. It made my job easier. I laid out the procedure. No recriminations. Just hard facts. The money, the time frame, the paperwork hassle with the state. Days or weeks, but as soon as possible if I made a call early Monday. Too late to make it that afternoon. Regional offices close at four in the afternoon.

And it'd be a thousand dollars or so.

During those years, people would come into the office thinking it's going to take a couple hundred bucks to get out of that sort of jam. They were wrong, and I was the guy who told them that the booze and the ticket meant they were going to be spending a whole lot of time and even more money trapped in an uncaring bureaucracy.

"Oh, God," she said. "I don't have it, and I've got to have my license by Monday so I can get to work."

The woman was thirty, I guessed, but I can't recall her face. I remember she was slender, with dark hair down to her shoulders, dressed in jeans and a denim jacket. Ask me now, and I'd say she was hard-used, too diffident and too beaten down for a woman so young. But that's hindsight, I know. I wished I had looked close into her eyes. Connected with her. Despair is difficult to hide. Maybe one word from me would have deflected the demon bearing down on her.

Did she blink or sigh when I outlined the solution? Did her shoulders slump? I can't remember. I was too wrapped up in my world, closed off to any emotions but my own. I did not care because I had not caused the problem. I could not care because there was nothing I could do to solve the problem. I did not care, but I didn't realize it was going to be car insurance or a bullet. I only learned about it later when the police called to trace her steps.

Surely the mess surrounding her DWI conviction wasn't the only thing that convinced her that a bullet in the brain beat battling through one more of life's messes. Marital friction, loss of job, alcoholism? It had to be something more than a couple of years' worth of high premiums and administrative paperwork.

You've got to be so far down in the dumps that you've lost the map to reality to choose suicide over higher insurance premiums.

When I heard the news, I wondered why so many of us are eager to take the express exit. We make a lot of noise about loving life, but the life we love isn't the life we can expect to live.

We are married to reality, for better or worse, in sickness and in health, and yet we expect to escape pain and adversity in spite of carelessness or stupidity or simple bad luck. And then, when life turns sour, there are those who celebrate the sanctity of self by turning their backs on the world rather than seeking solace somewhere.

When I remember the number of times I have thought about suicide, I think about the woman in my office, the early evening light dwindling through the door behind her. I wonder if she would have found a solution different from a bullet if she had gone home to someone who said, "Ah, baby, don't worry. We can work this mess out."

There was the police investigation. And the newspaper headlines.

And the talk around town. Society doesn't like it if you kill yourself because you're depressed. The city police called me the next day wanting me to relate the circumstances of my meeting with the woman.

"We need to investigate this thoroughly to rule out foul play," the officer said when he dropped by the office later that afternoon.

"Sure," I said. I recited the conversation from the previous day.

Inside I felt cold. And a tinge of guilt. Deep inside I wondered . . . what? The effect of my words? Why I hadn't paid closer attention? Could I have been the one to keep her finger off the trigger?

The officer asked for additional details, but I only knew that we all are mysteries to one another, that we are pulled one way or another by the things we tell ourselves, that occasionally we seek to quiet the voices with a drink or a pill, and that sometimes the best we can do is cling to each other in the night and shut our eyes against the dark. And sometimes even that doesn't work.

I told the officer something like that, but it didn't change anything.

I think of that woman whenever I read about the ongoing public discussion of assisted suicide. The discussion is reaching the stage when it's acceptable to ask for the seal of approval if you're depressed. Life will kill you but, if you're in a hurry, you can get help in punching your ticket out of this world.

Of course, there's one catch if you're hot to leave because you're depressed: you also must have a disability or a terminal disease.

Admittedly, the effort to approve assisted suicide has been minimally successful so far, concentrated mostly in Europe and in isolated places in the United States. Nevertheless, a significant element of society works for its approval by lobbying legislators and the media about the so-called right to die.

As if we had any choice . . .

Those rallying for a quick and painless death apparently think free will cannot provide a sufficiently lethal weapon. The advocates believe there should be a state-sponsored and regulated process, all in the name of humane objectivism. According to these advocates, physician-assisted suicide services should be a kindness reserved for the dying and the disabled. But that's not the whole truth, if you think about it carefully. A person must be terminally ill or permanently disabled—and despondent and depressed.

The melancholy lady who sat across from me on that soft fall afternoon long ago would have been denied the easy out however fervently she wanted off this earth. Assisted suicide proponents do not think people should be killing themselves simply because they've had a bad day at the office, their credit cards are toast, or their husband is in Cancún with his secretary.

Puzzling, isn't it? Depression is considered treatable, but only if you're perfectly healthy physically. Otherwise, depression is a valid reason for killing yourself.

Of course, there's a certain Swiftian logic behind physician-assisted suicide laws. Early exits tighten up cost overruns for HMOs and eliminate demands for hospital and long-term-care bed space. Swift might even have suggested that encouraging people with disabilities to choose death over access and accommodation would also lower educational and vocational budgets, eliminate the need for attendant care programs and other social services, and reduce demands for more ramps and curb cuts.

National right-to-die organizations like the Hemlock Society lobby for assisted suicide in the name of alleviating suffering in the face of terminal illness or disability. But even if a person's disability is a terminal illness, why should the solution be self-murder? Why cannot people at the end of their lives expect compassion and kindness, a chance to make peace with the world, without being pressured into considering self-destruction because of the fear of pain and discomfort? Why should the terminally ill give up the days allotted to them because it inconveniences others who should offer humane and supportive treatment?

But it is after we consider the influence of disability that the brutal logic rationalizing death over life is twisted to the point of disconnection.

According to a paper published by Stephen J. Taylor at the Center on Human Policy, Syracuse University, in April 2000, Dr. Jack Kevorkian, operating at the fringe of the right-to-die movement, "has publicly acknowledged helping at least 130 people to die by assisted suicide." A majority were women. Many were people coping with multiple sclerosis, a disease for which symptoms can be managed. One victim said she had chronic fatigue syndrome. Another claimed unspecified abdominal and pelvic pain. One woman, with a history of alcohol and drug abuse as well as emotional problems, had been diagnosed with multiple sclerosis, but an autopsy revealed no sign of the disease.

Tell me these men and women were not depressed. Tell me they were not living in despair because of ineffective medical care, or because of draconian laws restricting pain-alleviating drugs, or because of nonexistent counseling.

And then tell me that people with disabilities would not prefer access, accommodation, and sophisticated medical treatment to a needle and a lethal dose of narcotics.

19

I no longer believe I will kill myself, but I think I know how I will die. I will drown. Not for me the cancer or heart disease so common within my family. Not for me a clogged artery or stroke or lupus.

I will drown in my own mucus. My lungs will fill, and I will cease to be. I think I will be sorry.

I will drown and, as I fade, I will want time to tell those who love me not to grieve. For myself, I want to be sorry only for things undone, with only a few to count and those of no importance to anyone but me.

I play with this macabre resolution of my life—I say the words aloud to challenge the fear, to whistle past the graveyard of regret—because the disease of poliomyelitis left me to function for more than four decades with a mere one-fifth the lung capacity of an average adult male.

One side of my diaphragm is paralyzed and atrophied, and the other generates a cough reflex more befitting a kitten than a 150-pound man. A significant portion of the nerves firing the muscles of my ribcage and my back are damaged. I use the muscles of my stomach to inflate and deflate my lungs to their minimal capacity, and then only when I'm not using a respirator. Oddly enough, the workings of this damaged physical engine remain an involuntary process, for the body will forever seek to preserve itself.

I use a portable respirator for a majority of the day to prevent fatigue, and I sleep away each night at the end of that respirator's life-sustaining connection. I can breathe adequately away from my machine if I think about it not at all. I can breathe for eight hours or ten hours, or sometimes twelve or thirteen hours if I am having a good day. Then I tire, and I need—want, must have!—that assistance. If I think about it, if I acknowledge that the oxygen necessary for my engine to function is hard-won, I want assistance right away.

I survive this way because I cannot walk. There is little physical activity for my minimal respiratory function to sustain. I sit. I can move my hands and arms, but I can lift no weight greater than a few pounds. I am a quadriplegic, although a lucky one, because my arms and hands and random other muscles function well enough to keep me independent once I am lifted into my power wheelchair. Lucky also because I have sensory perceptions, feelings that permit pain signals to guard my legs and feet and buttocks—no pressure sores will become infected upon this body, thank you. Lucky because I no longer dream of running or of swimming or of lifting my wife in my arms and carrying her to our bed.

And lucky, most of all, because I find joy in being alive, in words and music, in the taste of fresh raw spinach with a touch of olive oil and balsamic vinegar, in the scent of flowers, in the flicker of film on screen, in the ideas leaping from book pages, in the playfulness and devotion of my dogs, and in the fragrance of my woman.

I believe in joy. I will it into my presence every day.

Toss me in bed, and I am as helpless as a turtle on its back in the middle of a highway. And as doomed. Toss me in bed, walk away, and close the door behind you, and I will die unless you return to aid me. Toss me in bed without my respirator, I will tire in a few hours, drift into a restless choking sleep, and die of respiratory insufficiency long before dehydration would kill me.

Please do not do such a thing. I am claustrophobic. I panic.

I love irony, but not this one: that the will to survive would act to hasten my death; that the fight-or-flight instinct would amplify into sheer panic; that because I can neither flee nor fight I would die even more quickly.

Panic, respiratory insufficiency, death: you can see why I never permit myself to be lifted into bed unless a telephone is handy.

My lungs may be waiting to kill me, but what is left of them is healthy. Of course, I am more than my lungs, even though a day does not pass that I do not think—*worry*—about them.

I imagine them as a pair of tricksters, playing fair as long as I keep watch, each of them working some secret magic. I think of my lungs as two sly and wizened old men, tottering about on withered crippled legs.

Because my lungs are waiting to kill me, because all remains well with them as long as I watch for their whispery reminders that they are tiring, I am constantly conscious of where I am in relation to the mechanical devices I need to keep me alive.

Breathing, you see, is an enterprise to be planned and monitored and regulated.

There are two machines, portable respirators. I keep one machine in my bedroom, and I carry the spare in our van. I do not want to be trapped away from home without access to positive pressure ventilation. The machine is a PLV-100, the size of a small tackle box, the case roughish metal painted a depressing institutional green. There are five dial knobs, four switches, four digital gauges, and one analog pressure dial. There is a single large hose marked "Patient Air" and two smaller hoses marked "Assist" and "Exhalation Valve" leading to the mask that clamps over my nose at night. The assist hose is dormant presently. I will not need it unless—until?—I descend to the point where I will require oxygen to be blended into the PLV-100's mechanically generated pressurized airflow—air, that flood of nitrogen, hydrogen, oxygen, and other ambient gases that keeps me alive at night and allows me to avoid fatigue during the day.

The machine looks like what it is, a medical device, and people stare at it obliquely if they happen to enter our bedroom. I once disliked people thinking me fragile—*I am a person with a disability! I am not ill!*—but then I remembered that I enjoy being alive, and I resolved never to hide the little green machine again.

After the iron lung, the rocking bed, the chest shell, and the pneumatic belt, I used nothing at all for twenty-five years. Over those two decades, I caught colds, influenza, and bronchial infections—the same disorders I believe may eventually start my journey to eternity. I survived these episodes by clearing my lungs and bronchial tubes by frog-breathing. It's simple. It's tricky. Take a quick gulp of sweet air, make a conscious effort to open the epiglottis valve at your bronchial tubes, and then force air down into your lungs by working your jaw and throat muscles. It can fill distressed lungs or gather in enough air to expel a peanut swallowed incorrectly or to generate a lung-clearing cough.

Frog-breathing, because from a viewer's perspective the workings of the throat mimic the appearance of a bullfrog when it sounds off to be recognized.

Frog-breathing, because it might keep me from croaking.

I prospered with frog-breathing at first, clearing my lungs or taking a deep breath. Now I prosper with the respirator, the latter having sufficient capacity to move far more air than an average human requires to generate a lung-clearing cough.

At night, I strap on a hose and mouth mask. The respiratory specialists refer to my choice of process for sleeping as noninvasive ventilation, a modern boon that can often substitute for a tracheotomy and its related problems. My initial nighttime ventilation masks were simple triangles of plastic with a rubber bushing seal. They were held against my nostrils by stretchable straps. When I first began to sleep with the mask and respirator, I had trouble. Wrongly positioned or too tightly bound, the mask's flexing movement would cut my nose. I would often go to work with a bandage across the bridge of my nose. I did not care. I would have embraced blood on my nose every morning of the remainder of my days in exchange for my life. I soon learned to fold a piece of tissue and place it across the bridge of my nose. That was in 1987. Today the masks are more comfortable. The present model is green, not institutional green but rather a darker forest green, nearly glowing with luminescent depth because of the sea-blue-green gel filling the cushions which rest against my face.

It is smaller than the oxygen masks worn by military pilots or mountaineers scaling Everest. It does not extend below my mouth. Even so, it is difficult to watch television from behind the mask, for I cannot wear my glasses. I do not care. Its straps once impressed oddly shaped paths in my hair. I did not care. I bought barber's clippers and trimmed my thinning, receding hair down to stubble.

I love the mask and the machine that fills it with blessed air fifteen times a minute, 1200 cubic centimeters of God's oxygen mixed with other harmless gases. A few precious cubic centimeters will spill from around the mask's imperfect seal against my face, but the rest—the *vital* in "vital capacity," that capricious measurement of intake and output—will fill my lungs with one more of a finite number of life-sustaining balloons of air.

I love my mask, even though a longtime friend, one who had polio a few years before me but does not yet need ventilation assistance, once saw a deep cut across my nose and said, "Oh, God, I don't see how you stand it."

I laughed. What's not to stand? I suck sustenance from the mask—it is my connection to life. And I find joy in life. I intend to live every second I can. I consider myself lucky, mostly because I believe I understand enough about the damage inflicted on me that I also comprehend how to keep myself alive. I know I'm lucky, really, because I can sometimes forget about oxygen and breathlessness, blood gases and the struggles of respiratory insufficiency, atrophied muscles and the imperfect technology that compensates for them.

I also fight the end I fear by avoiding crowds during flu season. I stay away from friends who are infected. And I plan to battle every random common cold before it degenerates into a virulent bronchitis. I am ever wary, guarding against intrusions across the frontier of disaster, storing away compounds of pseudoephedrine hydrochloride for the day my sinuses begin to fill, demanding that my physician allow me to keep a course of antibiotics handy in my medicine cabinet. I line up each year for influenza and pneumonia vaccines, hoping to outwit the always-evolving viral or bacterial fiends fighting modern pharmaceuticals.

I do not think I will give up easily. I will resist the microbes that breed with brute indifference, and I will fight because I love life.

Nevertheless, I believe I will drown.

20

I use a urinal. I carry my chamberpot in a book bag, a soft tan-colored burlap disguise. When I'm rolling through the free world, I hook the bag on the back of my wheelchair. I sometimes wonder if people recognize its shape, this pot I pee in, this distinctive square bottle with a round neck, at a glance familiar to almost everyone.

The book bag, my pot's camouflage, is marked with the saying, "Outside of a dog, a book is a man's best friend. Inside of a dog, it's too dark to read."

That's Groucho Marx, who probably never used a urinal. Oh, perhaps on his death bed, but never like me, never as one of life's constant essentials, like shoes or a toothbrush. Although I have used my own private pee pot—not the same one, of course—for more than forty-five years, I cannot imagine, not even in my most sardonic mood, Groucho saying, "Outside of a toilet, a urinal is a man's best friend."

But it can be, if you can't stand up to pee.

I initially found myself extraordinarily self-conscious about the idea that I had to roll through the world carrying a pot to pee in, forced to expose my most intimate part to the breeze at inopportune times and places. Lately, I have reconciled with my awkward encumbrance, probably assisted by the fact that it is far easier today than even twenty years ago to find an accessible bathroom.

"Give a man a urinal," I once said to my wife, "and create an exhibitionist." We were parked waiting to enter a place where there would be no toilet available to me. She was watching for passersby while I sat in the back of the van filling my pot.

"Hurry up," she said, always eager to play the game. "I see a cop. You might get arrested."

If you're drafted as a soldier into the crip brigade, you'll learn to take every conceivable opportunity to void your bladder. First, it's central to good health. The consumption of liquid and the expulsion of waste is more important to people who are paralyzed than it is for people who get about on foot. Almost without exception, a person is assigned a urinal because of limited mobility. Limited mobility results in limited thirst. Limited thirst results in decreased hydration. Insufficient hydration results in damage to the body.

I realize now that's why the hospital staff in Springfield was so adamant about measuring urine output during the period I was in the iron lung. Dr. Cochran, my physician then, mandated a specific intake of liquid daily. Theoretically, I was supposed to match that in output. Measure in, measure out—1000cc in and at least 1000cc out—continued throughout my stay in the hospital and the rehabilitation center.

Hydration for health. Good for me. Good for you.

Give a man a urinal and turn him loose to fend for himself, and he thinks differently. He thinks the way I have thought during a good portion of my nearly fifty wheelchair years.

"Where in the world can I find a private place to pee, and where can I empty the urinal when I'm finished?"

As I began to learn how to use a urinal in the real world, that meant hydration for health carried a caveat—hydration according to the availability of privacy. Early on, I despised announcing my intention and then seeking a place to use the urinal. I wanted privacy. I never developed the ability to ask for a towel or take my jacket and cover my groin, unzip, and sprinkle the urinal while people stood around pretending not to watch.

I saw an old man do that once, pee in public. I had moved to sit among a group of lawn-chair spectators at the end of a rodeo grandstand, and the old man was nearby. His wife handed him urinal and towel. He did his business, and she took the jar and walked under the grandstand to pour the waste in the dirt.

Cotton was the old fellow's name, and I knew him through my father. He'd been a blacksmith, a man strong enough to pound shoes onto horses' hooves while the beasts leaned against him. Now he had cancer, weighed little more than three or four good saddles, and didn't care what anyone thought.

For my part, I wheeled out in the parking lot that evening when I needed to pee. I found shelter between parked cars, did my business, and leaned over to baptize the gray-brown talcum powder dust. I thought about Cotton as I did, glad for my privacy, and I wondered how bottomless the pit of pain needed to be before I would recognize the urinal as something other than an emblem of antinormalcy.

Of course, that was in the 1960s. There were few accessible bathrooms anywhere, let alone in rural areas. In fact, accessibility of almost every type was utopian fiction, something for the future, when wheelchairs would be as antiquated as outhouses at a rodeo arena.

But today, for me, the issue of the urinal remains. I intermittently struggle with the idea that I must carry a pot to pee in, and the struggle forces me to turn my back on the misapprehension that others find the process—the device? me?—dirty.

Actually, urine is sterile, at least to you when it exits your body. You won't get sick if you pee on yourself. A urinal can be dirty, of course, what with the build-up of bacteria on waste remnants in an unwashed pot. I try to keep mine clean. I rinse it after use, and every evening I douse it with antiseptic liquid soap and let it stand overnight.

But you don't like my pee, and I don't like yours. That's normal. We are invariably reminded of that when we visit a public restroom and find ourselves greeted with the unmistakable fragrance of earthy, acidic liquid waste mixed with the brassy clang of industrial cleanser. That's hardly perfumed air.

Few of us discuss affairs of the toilet, of course. I can only speak for men, we creatures with two heads, we of soft egos that flop loosely toward the porcelain walls of restroom facilities. And, more particularly, for men who are disabled.

Men's restrooms are redolent with the stink of men, and all that is blood-simple and venereal about the gender. I do not fool myself, though. Cripples are asexual. I am no challenge to anyone's illusions of his own manhood. Nevertheless, I enter to stares when I bulldoze my wheelchair through the door of a public restroom. I feel eyes following me as I choose the stand-and-deliver farthest from the door. I slip down in my chair. Zip open my pants. If someone is standing at the next urinal, he can look down on my accomplishments, look for the genie in the bottle. I dump my waste and then seek out a liquid soap dispenser so that I can disguise any odor as I continue the day's journey. Groucho opens his bag, and we leave.

Nowadays, I keep a urinal at home, one at our cabin retreat, and one in our vehicle for Groucho to fetch along in his bag. I cannot tell you when my attitude toward my bottle, my urinal, my catcher-of-the-pee began to evolve toward acceptance, and then moved beyond, even though I still refuse to carry one in the open.

Perhaps there is even something right and logical about capturing liquid waste in a jar. When I urinate into the bottle and lift up the life-warmth encased within, seeking the "me" that is suspended in liquid, I think about what will become of me—the creature who is now suspended in flesh but one day will be ashes and dust. I feel the reality of it most when I am outdoors. I always search for a private place to return to the world what I cannot use—a storm drain, a link to the sea, or an isolated grassy spot to baptize.

No one has ever challenged me. Most, if they notice the urinal, turn away.

. . . .

On this midwinter's day in the sixth decade of my life, I have eaten a peanut butter and honey sandwich on pumpernickel bread for breakfast, a banana at midmorning, a can of butter beans drizzled with soy sauce in the early afternoon, and three ears of corn on the cob in the evening. I have downed one glass of water, a small glass of wine, and five enormous beer steins filled with hot tea.

One of the first cold, hard facts I learned in Omaha was that a good part of the rest of my life as a crip—at least in the mornings—would be spent flying a bedpan. I didn't really learn to hate bedpans then. Instead I worried most about the unending cycle of constipation, stomachaches, and cramping bowels. These were the day-long, night-rendering symptoms of a reluctant metabolism suddenly switched from an active teenager to a dormant near-skeleton—pain, nausea, and cramping, aggravated by the idea that relief could only be achieved if I cried out for help to clamp a hard metal device to my fanny.

Polio, unlike a traumatic spinal injury, normally leaves a person with bowel and bladder control. But when a person has been paralyzed to the extent that standing or shifting from wheelchair to toilet is not possible, the best alternative becomes an accessible bathroom and a commode chair. In my parents' farm house, the bathroom was filled with tub, toilet, and sink. There was no need for a commode chair because my parents could not afford to build a bathroom big enough to accommodate it. Thus, upon my release into the world, the choice became a bedpan or a diaper.

What I really needed was a lesson from a swami. If a guru can stop bleeding, change heart rates, and slow breathing patterns, I suspect one might have been able to teach my body to float above a bedpan and expel waste through mind control—or even sublimate discomfort to the extent that the metal bedpan became a mere bed of nails. Better yet, the swami could have taught me to eat correctly and hydrate properly, something neither the hospital, the physicians, nor the rehabilitation specialists mentioned.

What some health professional should have made sure I learned was not to obsess over this thing rarely discussed, this expulsion of dark, smelly waste, the shame of which plagues so many people with mobility disabilities. Of course, I realized something had to give, so to speak, when I would ride for days without a bowel movement, but I worried constantly because I understood my body had a mind of its own. I knew it did not plan to notify me or schedule my guts to expel a mess only when there was someone nearby who had the time, strength, and patience to lift me onto a bedpan.

As a boy, I had loved all the wrong foods for the right reasons—taste, sensual gratification. Liverwurst on white bread sandwiches, but only if they were liberally slathered in French's bright yellow mustard. Candy, particularly Snickers and Baby Ruth bars. And the small chilled bottles of Coca-Cola so common in the 1950s. I ate hamburgers by the handful and hot dogs by the yard, and I hated green and yellow vegetables. Pre–Julia Child, especially among American country cooks, such vegetables were simply boiled and ladled in clumps onto dinner plates. Steam was for ironing clothes.

Of course, the level of my physical activity decreased drastically after polio. But when I returned home to my mother's cooking, there was no parallel reduction in appetite for all the things that should be enjoyed in moderation.

No more school athlete. No more farm boy, up at dawn to milk dairy cows and then home after sports practice to milk once more and feed cattle again. No more hay hauling. No more summer work on a milk truck route. No more multiple pieces of fried chicken with a pile of mashed potatoes and gravy. No more chili and two sandwiches for lunch. No more candy, milkshakes, and Coca-Cola.

No more access to a nearby toilet whenever the urge struck.

Canned in the iron lung, I had become a withering, wasting mass of insecurities, apprehensions, and depression. The dessicated body housed in the great machine needed minimal fuel, and minimal fuel produces little waste. I don't remember refusing to eat. I simply didn't care. I remember spoons pressed against my lips, but I did not take them. I was not hungry.

The doctors said, "Give him anything he wants." Nurses had offered treats. My mother brought food from home. Still I did not eat. My body, I think, was waiting for my spirit to make up its mind to live. The spirit decides, and the spirit may not always concede the power of its decision to the rational self.

Days passed in the hospital, and I continued to lose weight. The doctor finally said, "I'm going to prescribe an appetizer cocktail—a stimulant."

The concoction, prim in its little paper shot glass on the nurse's medication tray, contained alcohol, I suspect, but it was no sophisticated manhattan or playful mimosa. It tasted almost like a vile brew of castor oil, grease, and vodka. I drank it straight from the paper cup in one viscous gulp, three times a day, for weeks, cringing as it burned its way into my stomach. I continued to nibble at food in response to threats and persuasions. And then the nurses discovered the appetite stimulant was supposed to be mixed with something like orange juice or milk to disguise its taste.

Did it begin to work after they corrected the dosing mechanism? I only know I began to eat.

First, a few spoonfuls of mashed potatoes or green beans. Next, more nibbles from other parts of the day's hospital fare. When my mother was able to make the trip to the hospital, usually every other day, she would stop by the cafeteria and bring me a milkshake or a grilled cheese sandwich, made with dill pickles embedded in the gooey cheese still warm enough to ooze from the edge of the bread.

Matter can be converted to energy, but we know that the process is not perfect in the case of our biological engines. A body burns fuel in the form of food, and then the leftovers from that conversion become urine and feces. And so, after I began to eat tiny but regular meals, the nurses and aides attempted to create a schedule for me to expel such waste. Each morning before my sponge bath, I would be turned onto a bedpan, thus introducing me to the hard metal throne I was to use every morning for years.

"Turned onto" meant I became lever to the bedpan's fulcrum, which was the simplest part of the process. I was soon to discover that human beings sit upright on toilets to expel solid waste for a particular reason—the process works best in a position where it's aided by gravity. The second complication was that my trunk muscles were almost useless. I could grunt, but all that, in the words of Macbeth's lament, was "sound and fury signifying nothing."

I was to use a bedpan throughout the time I lived in the iron lung, both in Springfield and in Omaha, and I used it for several years after, right up until Everest & Jennings built—and I discovered I could use—a commode chair. Granted, once free of the iron lung, I could ask that the rocking bed, and the hospital bed I used after that device, be cranked upward to perhaps thirty or forty degrees above horizontal, but even that significant increase in angle did little to make the bedpan less painful or more useful.

I sat, but I seldom shat.

But I was lucky in my search for an equilibrium between fuel and waste, the process so critical to good health for people who are paralyzed. Lucky, first, because even though it was painful and awkward, I could at least void waste by natural means rather than relying on medical intervention, and second, because the assorted physicians who monitored my journey refused to give me laxatives or stool softeners, except in one or two emergency cases.

"They're addictive," said one doctor, "and hard on the bowels."

Like most people, I accepted some medical advice and rejected other suggestions. I did learn that on the occasions when I resorted to a laxative that the chemicals functioned unpredictably. It is one of life's uglier and messier frustrations to feel bowels painfully cramping and have no chance to tend to their demands. The frustration is amplified if a wheelchair is involved, and there is no toilet readily available, and no assistance, and there becomes no recourse but to sit in the foul mess so violently, and reluctantly, expelled.

I was lucky also because once free of the hospital and rehabilitation center, once home to my mother's cooking, once able to enjoy a restaurant on occasion, I began to eat, and then eat more. My strength began to return, and my immune system and metabolism began to regulate themselves toward some semblance of a new normalcy.

I followed a diet limiting calcium-rich food at first, one designed to prevent the formation of kidney stones, which were the bane of a sedentary life according to the staff at the rehabilitation center. But my mother's cooking won out, and I ate anything offered. And then more. Never so much as to become obese or even overweight, but enough of all the wrong things, taking too many steps down the wrong road to regularity. I ate for sensuous pleasure, one of the last pleasures left to me other than an afternoon in the sun or a night of erotic dreams. I ate all the wrong things for all the right reasons, except one, perhaps.

It was good that I wanted to eat and that I ate, but it was bad that my return home to my mother's familiar cooking encouraged me to believe an untruth—that not everything had changed. Of course, I needed to gain weight to build strength, but I did not eat the things necessary to allow me to gain weight properly. I had been constipated in the hospital when I ate nearly nothing or little more than nothing, and now I was constipated at home when I was hungry and had access to the favorite foods that would satisfy my hunger.

Constipated first for days, then for months, and finally for years, able to expel only little tidbits of waste.

And that I accomplished by grunting myself into exhaustion and inflicting crushing pressure on my lower abdomen with my hands and elbows. I rode my chair for a decade, my gut overstuffed, cramped, bloated, nauseous. In that period—too ignorant to eat correctly or to drink adequate amounts of liquid—I managed to avoid instances as trivial as fouling my pants, at least not on a regular basis and rarely in public, or as serious as an impacted bowel, which might have killed me.

Gradually, I have learned to survive, eating less as each year spends itself, marveling at the apparently minimal amounts of nourishment a mature human body needs. That I am healthy after almost fifty years of using a wheelchair—my weight under control, my metabolism slowing but harmonizing itself to a vegetarian diet without rebellion—has come about without calculation on my part.

I had no reason to stop eating meat in my late fifties. I simply stopped for a few days and found myself feeling better. I am no eat-right evangelist, but nonetheless a wise person recognizes that age slows metabolism. Of course, my own had already dwindled to sloth-level because of an inability to walk. That's why we became good friends, my bowel and me. When I paid little attention, he became a snake who let me down in public, although no doubt fewer times than I deserved. Now I treat him more kindly than I once did, and we give into one another's requirements, cooperating to seize a chance each day to rid ourselves of solid waste.

Admittedly, I am a slow learner, and so I was a reluctant partner at first. "Eat prunes," my mother said.

I simply added prunes and kept on enjoying barbecue, spaghetti with extra meatballs, and two scoops of coffee ice cream on devil's food cake. Good enough, but as I began to comprehend that I was eating too much and gaining weight, I changed my diet to what it should have been years ago.

Weight? Even if a man cannot stand on a scale, peek between his feet, and watch the numbers spin upward, he learns a dietary lesson when he's forced to buy pants in a larger waist size. No guesswork necessary.

Now I eat fresh fruit. I eat beans and corn. I eat eggs and whole grain bread and whole grain cereal. I eat spinach, broccoli, tomatoes, onions, avocados, soy beans, sunflower kernels, and peanut butter. I eat no meat, not even fish or chicken. And I eat all that sparingly, chased with two or three liters of fluid daily.

By adjustment and experimentation, by dispassion and discipline, and by stoicism and apathy, I have learned to eat to live rather than live to eat.

By some combination of divine grace, rugged genes, and unwitting choices, I have been able to avoid any illnesses related to kidneys, bladder, or bowels—the trio so often the bane of wheelchair riders. I am spare like my father, a grateful inheritance, and find it relatively easy to stay that way. Too many pounds would adversely influence my vital capacity, because my weakened lungs would be forced to work against the bulk of an oversize belly.

I am a quadriplegic, more or less, but I still have sensory perceptions. Thus, I am not subject to pressure sores or other health concerns resulting from the inability to discern other vital bodily processes.

I had polio, but the random nature of the damage the disease inflicted upon my nervous system does not require me to use a catheter or a colostomy bag.

I am male, the half of humanity whose physiology allows for simple, direct liquid waste disposal, even from a wheelchair.

And I am blessed with a constitution and a metabolism that respond to the power of will.

I am a lucky man.

21

I have worn out seven wheelchairs in forty-plus years. More accurately, I've worn out six, and I have been worn out by one. None of them were equipped with odometers. I can't tell you the number of miles I've ridden. I can only say it's been a long, strange journey.

The first two were me-powered—me, grasping the offset wheel rims, pushing this way, pulling that, sometimes simultaneously, to spin and rotate, move forward and back up, and stall and flounder on rough or uneven surfaces.

The last five have been driven by battery-powered electric motors. Electric chairs. Electric chairs put away criminals, and when I thought I was being punished by disability, that's what I called my power chair, the first one, my *Electric Chair*. Back then all the artistic energy I had left after conjuring up fantasies of walking I devoted to crafting dramas of self-pity.

I was thirty years old and had gained back all that was to be left of me when my mother suggested that a power chair would further liberate me. I felt strong, and so I saw no need to change. My father agreed with me. "You don't want to mess with that. You'll never get any exercise." My father was the sort of man who'd fight you until he couldn't get off the ground, and then he'd bite your ankle.

Hand-powering a chair, accomplished by grasping a metal outrigger rim attached to the rear tires and then pushing and pulling over rough ground and smooth ground, deep carpet and wood floors, was exercise, no doubt about it, and it helped keep my weight under control.

During that period of my life, I had tired of the insurance business and the longer commute from outside Aurora, where we moved in 1972, so I had taken a job offer from a small town radio station. It was work no one wanted—scheduling commercials and news and keeping program logs demanded by the Federal Communications Commission. In the jargon of that business, I was the traffic manager. It didn't pay much, but it did earn attention from the station's salespeople, the manager, the purchasers of air time, and the occasional correspondent from FCC. All of them had different ideas about who should share the minutes allotted for commercials every hour of broadcast, how many public service announcements were to be aired, and which church broadcast should get the best slot. The four previous people who had worked the job had lasted no more than six months each.

In spite of the regional manager telling the local manager, "Don't hire a guy in a wheelchair. He'll be out sick too much," I earned the job because the local guy liked my sense of humor and was impressed that I knew without being told that competitive car dealers' commercials shouldn't be run back to back. I stayed for four years. The little 500-watt station was part of a small chain of broadcast stations owned by a man from Texas. He kept a constant eye on costs in order to boost the profit margin, and so, as I became more familiar with what was necessary to keep the place functioning, I had more work shuffled to my desk—writing commercials and news, helping with promotions, and even appearing on the air occasionally. It was hectic work. After a day of racing around the halls of the studio, I was ready for a good night's sleep.

I was strong, I had calluses on hands that stayed dirty—think about the results of an inadvertent spin through dog poop or food spilled on the floor—but I wasn't a wheelchair athlete, one of those people crashing through the Paralymics or burning up a marathon.

Damn, I thought back then, if I was that strong I'd get out of the chair and walk on my hands. I mistakenly—enviously?—viewed wheelchair athletes as disability impostors. They appeared to be bizarre centaurs—from belly up, weight-lifting pro wrestlers, and from belly-down, the skeletal hips and legs of long-term prisoners of war.

Actually, it's an image I still hold, dual-bodied men and women, half superhero, half crip. The only tolerable thing about my continued slippery grasp on *Who really has earned the right to be labeled as a person with a disability?* is that my resentment of long ago has evolved into practical admiration.

My mother won out, as was often the case with my father and always the case with me. "You're going to be able to do so much more without help, Gary," she said.

A few days later, we piled in the van and drove to a shop in Springfield.

Back then, I was a crip all over, starting at the brain. And I nearly made my situation worse by breaking my neck the first time I got into a power chair.

Crip equipment is high-dollar stuff, and I expected a nice building and trendy decor when I went shopping for my first power chair, but the guy running the place wasn't investing his income in capital improvements. The Victorian-era merchant building backing up to a set of railroad tracks in north Springfield had a broad plank floor. When I took a test drive, I sailed along quickly enough under battery power that I could feel the waves of imperfection in my fanny.

Butt surfing.

In spite of its antique appearance and the stand-offish attitude of the owner, Smithson Medical Equipment was a lucky choice, one found by pointing a finger at an advertisement in the Yellow Pages. That's because the store employed an empathetic and talented wheelchair technician named Ben. Mr. Smithson was prosperous, well dressed, and distant. Ben was a slender, oddly shaped man my age, distinguished by having more tattoos than teeth. Smithson watched over the profits. Ben watched over the customers.

"Slowly now," Ben said as I goosed that first power chair up the folding door ramp mounted on the side of my van.

Slowly I went, slowly enough, that is, until the front of the chair crested the apex of the ramp. I should have let up on the power immediately, but I didn't, and the chair took a leap, and I forgot to duck. "Crack!" My head hit the top of the door frame hard enough to make me nauseous.

Not a good beginning, all in all, but not enough to deter me. Within a few days, I grew to love the freedom offered by my electric legs. Freedom simply in being able to cover yards—miles!—of distance without aid. Freedom at my fingertips. Freedom in sensation, stimulation, and spectacle. Freedom in a world expanded and open for exploration.

My first three power chairs were belt and pulley affairs. That comes to mind primarily because I once used one to accidentally kill a pure-bred Himalayan kitten. I was preparing supper, and I didn't notice that the little creature had climbed the rear drive tire. I spun off to open the refrigerator. The kitten—Mouse was her name—clung to the tire as it moved, and she quickly circled around to meet her doom, pinched between belt and wheel hard enough to break her neck.

I have also done lesser damage with power wheelchairs. Nicks, scratches, and scars on desks and other pieces of furniture, plus chunks of plaster knocked from hallway walls and wood trim peeled from doorway openings. I won't bother to list the dozens of store displays, especially since merchants prefer plentiful goods in sight on wide aisles crowded to near inaccessibility by crammed displays. We can also count a snapped bone in my right ankle—*Who cares? I can't walk anyway*—bruises and cuts on my knees too numerous to count—*They'll heal*—and two dislocated knuckles in my left index finger—*I can still type.*

Actually, "power" chair is a better description than electric chair when we consider the mass-in-motion kinetic energy of a 150-pound man riding 200 pounds of steel frame and lead batteries. There were also other imperfections in that first chair. It had an inherent electro-mechanical defect that taught me to pay strict attention to where it was and what it might do.

A product of Everest & Jennings, then the premier manufacturer of wheelchairs in the USA, the chair had the tendency to start up on its own and move off at high speed in a random direction. Never predictable, it often buzzed off several feet before I could grab the control. More than once I was jerked out of a reading session or some other benign activity—two hands on my book or otherwise far from the control stick—and flung into the nearest wall or piece of furniture.

"Hey, Ben," I said to the technician on a trip to the store for new tires. "Have you heard of one of these things starting up out of the blue and shooting off by itself?"

"Yeah," he replied. "Be careful. The factory thinks it may be caused by static build-up tripping the mechanical relays. There's this old gal on the other side of town, well, it happened to her, and she sailed plumb off her patio."

That got my attention. I thought for a while, and then I remembered seeing gasoline tanker trucks dragging pieces of chain. Drivers believed the dangling metal created a static discharge path to ground, thus lessening the chance of fire and explosion. When we got home, I found an old section of dog collar and created my own ground loop. It may have helped. It may not have. I took no chances. When I stopped for any length of time, I tried my best to remember to turn off the power switch. I had that chair three or four years. I got a bruised foot or knee occasionally when the ghost in the machine wanted to play a trick, but I was never launched from a patio.

When I was ready for another chair, E & J was still the major player in the disability equipment market, and, like most people when dealing with all that is vital in life, I stuck with what worked. By then, the company had updated the control system, and the Let's go for a ride now! problem was no more.

That first power chair cost me a bit more than $1,100. It was the top of the line. The next was $1,800. Then I remember one at almost $4,000. Those three were all E & J machines. All looked like a standard wheelchair of that era: big bicycle-style wheels at the rear, caster wheels in front, a metal framework rigged to hold a sling seat and sling back. But when I was ready to replace the third chair, I learned

E & J was no more, or at least not a major presence in dealer display rooms. And it is that next power wheelchair, my fourth and the first of another brand, a beast that could not be rode, that truly sticks in my memory—and not because I spent $7,400 on it.

I had worn out my latest E & J, and the medical equipment dealers were pushing products made by a company called Invacare. To me, the company name seemed nothing more than a Madison Avenue amalgamation, an ugly stepchild created from the ill-considered marriage of "invalid" and "care," although I was later told the in stood for innovation. My thought was to simply call it Cripmobile and be done with it.

By this time, Ben, the technician, had moved to another shop. I followed him. The owner of Brass Medical Equipment rolled out the new model. Mr. Brass said, "This is the one you want, Gary."

Despite the name, he was right. I wanted that Invacare, the company's Action model. I desired that particular model because it looked nothing like a traditional wheelchair. It had the appearance of a nifty bucket seat taken from a sports car and mounted atop a sleek plastic box.

I bought it. After using it a day or two, I was surprised and confused to realize it was awkward and uncomfortable. Days passed, and my feeling that I had jumped on the wrong bandwagon deepened, even though the new chair ran faster and felt more stable. I began to hate it, and to regret shelling out the money, even though it was gear-driven and thus incapable of garroting innocent kittens. I hated it because it was unpleasant to sit in and cumbersome to maneuver.

I did more damage with that chair during the eighteen months I used it than I had accomplished with all three previous power chairs. For more than a dozen years, I had powered myself through houses and offices, up slopes and across lawns, through businesses and down sidewalks. A nick here, a notch there, of course, but not every day. Now, saddled up and riding my dream chair, I found myself ricocheting between apologies and curses because the damnable thing never seemed to go where I pointed it.

And then there was the question of my health.

I believe in pain. Pain warns. Pain protects. Pain teaches. But that chair inflicted pain without profit. My hips and back began to hurt so much that I could not spend a full day in it. Brass called the factory, and experts came to consult with me, but the only way I could find relief was to corkscrew my back into a misaligned mess, which provided relief for my hips and legs but did nothing for my posture. I changed seat cushions. No relief. The back of the wheelchair was changed from a one-size-fits-all shape to one fitted to my frame, but the pain rolled on—a hot rod spiking out from my hips and searing up my spine. Constant pain, and I knew that was a signal for me to change something or I would end up with the problem I thought I had left at the rehabilitation center—pressure sores.

I had used all my previous power chairs for about three to five years before the squeaks, rattles, and hums reminded me that there are limits to mechanical service. Once to the bottom of a chair's tank, I bought another and put the old chair in my garage as a spare.

But not this one.

I hadn't used it for three months before I began to hope it would catch fire and burn. Without me in it, of course.

Alternately, I considered leaving it outside at night. Burglar bait, crime with built-in punishment.

But before two years had passed, riding in my worn old E & J spare chair as much as in the new Invacare, I gave up and decided frugality had its limits. I bought another chair.

The Iron Maiden went into the garage, fittingly hidden under two large garbage bags to shield it from dust. One day, looking at that source of so much discomfort, I realized I'll borrow money and buy something new before I park my ass in that piece of junk again. So I called the regional independent living center and offered it to them as a donation. I knew the center's mechanics could recondition it for use. And surely, I thought, there must be someone whose shape would allow them to fit into it without distress.

But I didn't let it go without a warning. When the volunteer loaded the beast into the center's van, I said, "That's the most uncomfortable chair I have used in thirty years. If someone complains that it hurts to ride in that thing, believe them, and then try it on someone else."

That chair, my one-out-of-seven mistake on wheels, had been only the second chair I had named. My first one, the one that set me on the road to near-independence, I called the Electric Chair, but when I jumped out of the Iron Maiden and into an Invacare Action Storm Series MKIV Ranger X, I decided to name my new companion in honor of its five-figure price—the Little Red Car.

Why do business again with the people who'd sold me a lemon? I returned to Invacare because it was the only company I could find that still offered a rear-wheel-drive power chair. Most of the new manufacturers entering the market and selling mobility devices to the last of the Greatest Generation and their offspring, the baby boomers aging early, were peddling front-wheel-drive units or six-wheel units with the drive wheels directly under the passenger. I tried one. I tried another. After more than a decade of being pushed to my destination, I couldn't drive a straight path on a perfectly level floor while being pulled along in the direction of choice. I moaned and whined, griped and cursed, and then I wrote another check to Invacare.

I ride in Little Red today, and I hope she will carry me home, as the old gospel song says. She is a remarkably spartan and utilitarian companion in spite of her complicated, oxymoronic official name.

I am Little Red. She is me. We are joined—cyborg—my little red chair and me, by a joystick control knob sticking up from an oddly shaped six-by-two-by-three inch metal box mounted near the left armrest.

According to legend, joystick is slang for a man's erect penis. That tactile description arises from the ribald attitude of aircraft pilot instructors and trainees learning to send their flying machines through three axes of space by using a vertical rod mounted between their legs.

My juvenile fantasy was to be a military pilot, a dream that stumbled over the teenage reality of myopia and died completely in the iron lung. All that remains of the long-ago fantasy is the joystick. And the one on my power chair resembles nothing so much as a black mushroom mounted upside down on the control box, a dark gnomish phallic symbol if it is one, the stunted remnant of a dream become nightmare.

I prefer my controls on the left side. "But aren't you right-handed?" asked Ben, when I bought my first chair. "If so, it's going to be more natural for you to point the chair using your right hand."

"Yeah, maybe. But if the control's on the left, I've got the hand I use most free to do other things. When you drive a standard shift, you point the car with your left hand, right?"

Ben swallowed any more advice and attached the control box on the left arm. From the instant I was lifted into its seat, I found the location a natural fit. Every chair I've purchased since has been controlled from the left side.

Little Red is comfortable. She's small, easily maneuverable, and rugged. I listen to her, and she has never left me stranded, not once in ten years or more. I cannot remember exactly how long she and I have been together. I only know I love her enough to have paid three times the cost of my first power chair to have her mechanical parts refurbished. And I've done that twice, each time responding to warnings murmuring deep in her gear bearings or yelps of pain screaming out from her spindles.

Little Red was once gone from Thursday afternoon until Monday morning, and I missed her each day, once so much that I accidentally ripped six feet of trim from a door after fumbling around with the inconsistencies of her ugly and recalcitrant substitute.

We are one, Little Red and me. Our neuropaths, hers electromechanical, mine electrochemical, connect where my thumb touches her joystick. Little Red cradles me, sweetly, soothingly, a sturdy girl, all power and promise.

I can't tell you the particulars of how we communicate. But here is one certain thing I know: I think; she moves.

I am hungry. I must fetch the makings of lunch, but there is no flight plan, no cockpit check-off list. There is simply the deed, each distinct movement necessary, accomplished. There is desire transmitted from brain to thumb to chair, complex instructions running a parallel path to the highway of my desire for an apple or a peanut butter sandwich.

I want to move from the computer desk to the refrigerator. I must back up slightly, then turn right ninety degrees, move eight or ten feet, rotate ninety degrees right again, grasp the handle of the refrigerator, back up three feet, and then brace my elbow to hold the door open. I can do that without thinking about it; I draft a flight plan from my subconscious by focusing on the desire for a destination. Ask me to describe the movements of my thumb, and the micrograms of pressure necessary to pinch the joystick against the third knuckle of my left index finger, and I cannot tell you.

A thoughtful person will never be *confined* to a wheelchair. I refuse to use the description. I will correct others who indulge in the fallacy. My chair takes me somewhere akin to the experience of the Six Million Dollar Man without the heroics. My chair enhances my physical capacity and thereby liberates me within my environment.

Once I moved into the town of Aurora, stout, reliable Little Red, plus a poncho and a down jacket, meant I could travel the mile and a half to work, on wheels, without asking someone to load me up and drive me there in my van. I could travel another mile past my office to the library. On the way home from work, I could stop by the supermarket.

With Little Red, I became a fixture in the town, a regular cruiser on its tree-lined streets. Streets? Yes, because before environmental issues and equal access to government services became a political and social movement, small towns in rural areas wrote zoning ordinances for two reasons: to promote industry and to protect influential neighborhoods. Rarely did they zone for accessibility, at least not until compelled to by the 1991 Americans with Disabilities Act. In the little town where I lived for fifteen years, there were few sidewalks in the residential areas and fewer curb cuts anywhere. I traveled on the streets.

"Somebody should give that guy a ticket," a local grouch told my employer. "He has no business running down the street in that thing."

But the police only waved from their patrol cars when they passed me.

I did see an officer stop and talk to another guy. That wheelchair user apparently had generated ill will among the town's animal lovers. I had noticed him, mostly at a distance, but I had never met the guy. I've always needed a reason other than the commonality of cripdom before I approach another person with a disability. This fellow had a super-crip chair, the sort of mobility device popular with paraplegics, especially those in athletic competition. Such chairs are little more than wheels connected by slings on which riders can sit. The lightweight rear wheels are cambered inward for maximum stability, and the tiny front casters are meant to minimize friction drag. It's a chair that can be hand-powered faster than the fastest standard motorized chair.

My rolling compatriot had shoulder-length hair, a patchy beard, and a wiry, loose-limbed frame. He appeared as if dressed in cast-offs, always blue jeans, but sometimes wearing only a sleeveless T-shirt when a jacket might be a better choice to shield him from the wind. His evident poverty and ramshackle appearance weren't the problem, though.

It was his dogs.

The beasts were pound mutts, I guessed. There were usually three of them, all relatively large animals, forty- or fifty-pound packages of canine in assorted shapes and colors. He tied them to the frame of his chair with what looked to be a homemade harness, and he convinced the beasts to pull him through the streets with a combination of yelling and an occasional pop with the remnants of a fishing pole. Not whippings with the fiberglass stick, at least not that I noticed, but rather a tap on a side or a nose to steer the pack, with him helping by using his free hand to provide drag on the wheel when he needed to make the turn.

"That greasy little son of a bitch is cruel to those dogs," a friend said to me. "Someone needs to slap him upside the head."

I didn't argue. I didn't know, in fact. People in the north use sled dogs, but, of course, these weren't sled dogs. Nevertheless, I had never heard them whine or yelp or seen them cower. They seemed fit enough. And for dogs, work can be play.

I never got close enough to the guy to make up my mind about the right and wrong of his choice. In fact, if I had tried to, I wouldn't have been able to catch him. My power chair can sail along at five to seven miles per hour. The dog chair left me in the dust.

I hope he didn't abuse his dogs, but I understood his need to move. To move faster. And further. I suppose he could have bought two or three Huskies or Malamutes or some other type bred for drafting. Perhaps that might have deflected some of the complaints from the town's animal lovers. But the choice of dogs, I suspect, was a matter of money—he apparently used dogs other people had thrown away.

Ask me now, these years later, and I will say I think he had learned what I had learned.

Sometimes living disabled is about asking someone for help, even if you have to swallow your misplaced self-respect and illusions of independence.

Other times it's looking on things with a cold eye and letting patience evolve into stoicism, if necessary, so that you can tolerate what you can't change.

And occasionally it's about hitching an old mongrel to necessity and moving on, no matter what anyone thinks.

22

On Labor Day, 2002, I received a phone call. "Go back to the TV, you fucking loser!" From three states east, a man found himself angry enough to telephone and tell me what he thought about an opinion piece I had written and sent to various newspapers. The essay he had read in the Cleveland *Plain Dealer* encouraged people to rethink their support of Jerry Lewis and his annual Muscular Dystrophy Telethon. My caller thought the multimillions of dollars Lewis raised with his theater of tragedy outweighed the comedian's lack of respect for people with disabilities.

At first, admittedly, the caller put me on the defensive. I have often debated whether the money Lewis raises accomplishes so much in practical medical research that it offsets the immeasurable social damage he inflicts. I've lived my adult life in a wheelchair, but I came late to disability activism and anti-telethon protests. As for Lewis himself, I had never connected personally to his maudlin pleas for money and creepy references to "my kids." Some of those kids were adults functioning in society.

Pity objectifies, dehumanizes, and denigrates. The stench of it makes me gag, even when it is not directed at me. Over the years, I found myself able to watch only a few minutes of Lewis's telethons or any other broadcast meant to generate dollars by displaying pain.

But then, after I had ridden through three decades in a wheelchair, I began writing about life as a person with a disability. I didn't write, really, to complain or to change things. I wrote because I found myself unsure of my place in the world, and I wanted to explore its boundaries. Then I came into contact with activists who maintained a long list of Jerry Lewis's actions and words. Reading the protestors' material left me believing that Lewis subconsciously felt disconnected from the humanity of the people he was supposed to be helping. I knew Lewis grew up following his father on the vaudeville circuit, and I understood that in that generation a person with a disability might be labeled a shut-in or an invalid. People with disabilities then were socially isolated because there were few opportunities for education and employment. I suspect the only people with disabilities Lewis saw during the first decades of his life were those working the freak-shows.

Most of us grow in awareness and sophistication, though, and our values change, and, if we're lucky and smart, it's for the better. Had this happened with Jerry Lewis? Most disability activists believed not. Lewis always seemed surprised when the criticism rained down after he'd popped off and used a description like "half-person" to characterize someone using a wheelchair.

And he rarely apologized.

"You don't want to be pitied because you're a cripple in a wheelchair, stay in your house." He said that once in a television interview when a reporter asked him about disability activists' protests. He meant it.

To some people, disability is leprosy; disability is the untouchable; disability always has its hand out for alms.

My parents were of Jerry's generation, a generation when a wheelchair signified mortality rather than mobility. "My son was crippled by polio," my father or mother might say, but it didn't bother me.

Rooted in Old English—*crypel*, to "creep"—cripple is one of those nouns that nearly perfectly illustrates its meaning. But my parents never called me a cripple. I was Gary, who happened to have been crippled by polio. I was their son, not a condition.

Good enough until I moved from the shelter of acceptance into the curiosity of the world. There the questions began.

"What put you in that chair?" people would ask when I was at work. "What's wrong with you?"

I tolerated the inquiries. More accurately, I politely deflected them, sometimes smiling and replying, "Nothing. I'm doing great today.

And how are you?" Somewhere in my natural emotional makeup I recognized that a person dances more gracefully through the world if he relies on good manners to fend off the boorish and the ignorant.

Nevertheless, I understood the questions demanded that I define myself. With an appearance so unlike that of the interrogator, I must be an alien species. Of course, I didn't need the questions to remind me that I was crippled, although when I found myself making a reference to my circumstances I toned down the description to more tractable words like "disabled" or "handicapped."

I was riding through the early stages of my evolution into Gary-on-wheels then—still throwing myself a pity party occasionally, no guest appearance by Jerry Lewis required—and the only descriptions I balked at were words and phrases like "confined to a wheelchair," "invalid," or "shut-in."

Soon, though, I began to notice a segment of people with disabilities who took words like "cripple" and threw them back into society's face. Great idea, that. Call yourself a crip, and you're certainly no longer *invalid*. You are . . . odd, eccentric, quixotic.

Shock has value, and I learned to appreciate it and employ it. A person with a disability who moves through a society of normals in spite of objections, warnings, or admonitions—in other words, a crip—has learned to watch eyes, to wait for signs of the unpalatable probing, for the graceless phrases being conjured up beneath sidelong glances, and for the forming resolution to voice what is best left unsaid.

And, if you work at being a crip long enough—an uppity crip, as one disability activist puts it—you assume a full-blown identity, one in which disability becomes an essential part of self.

I am Gimp. Hear me roar!

Each day I move about in the real world, each play staged and scene laid out, I enter as a novelty wrapped in a disability, a puzzle to be examined and probed, a visible alien in a virtual Roswell. I come equipped with the pejoratives, the cruel labels, the words that can cut, and I use those weapon words to seize control of any situation where prejudice might abound.

I use them because I have earned the right and because I've grown too jaded for social awkwardness and because others cannot. It's much like the black entertainer Chris Rock when he said, "Every time black people want to have a good time, niggers mess it up."

I like that attitude. I grew up on racially integrated military bases, across the country and around the world—Japan and France, California, Texas, and South Carolina. I spent my youth in schools and social environments with blacks, Hispanics, and Asians. Then I spent the early part of my adult life in small-town America, the Midwest of two-lane roads and little churches with white steeples, the land where few black Americans visited and fewer lived. And as I grew older, curious to expand my world, a time concurrent with my life journey aboard a wheelchair, I read the melancholy histories from the dark corners of our land, histories filled with lynchings, race riots, and Jim Crow laws.

And then I made a mistake. I made the sad assumption of equating the lack of access, the minimal employment opportunities, the social mindset that interpreted crips as less-than-complete persons with the blood-soaked saga of racial and ethnic discrimination. I constructed a confused and unsupportable analogy. I began to tell my parents and other people I trusted, "You know, being in a wheelchair is almost like being black."

Right. At least on the surface.

And wrong. Obscenely wrong.

A person of color and a person with a visible disability are both readily identifiable by appearance. That makes discrimination simpler. I felt excluded, true enough, because of perceptions based on my appearance, defined by Lewis and his ilk as a "half-person." But, of course, I had then and have now no understanding of the black experience in America, an experience that begin with slavery.

I am not a person of color. I am a person with a disability, and I've grown sufficiently to comprehend that the emotions I felt then were first generated by my isolation—enforced, but also voluntary to some degree—rather than by mindless prejudice of other people.

When I started to venture into the world and confront the unique prejudice generated by a visible disability, I learned that no one displayed angry prejudice toward crips and kicked them out of restaurants, or refused to let them in a state university, or denied them the right to vote.

And no one turned fire hoses on crips. Or lynched us. We were simply left to our families or shuffled off to institutions.

I felt ashamed about my feeble attempt to tap into an experience I could never share.

Before the Rehabilitation Act of 1973, people with disabilities were simply invisible. Discrimination reigned because of public ignorance and apathy. An ungodly number of crips had no option other than being warehoused in nursing homes and state institutions. Those free of confinement generally remained with families.

Sadly, many of us sat on porches, waited in family rooms and bedrooms, piddling with crossword puzzles, television, and paint-by-number kits; our peers moved out to colleges and universities and eventual employment. The Rehabilitation Act was the first step toward integration. The courageous crips had already struck out—who else to lobby and demonstrate for change?—and now the ambitious were able to take advantage.

Of course, the world of disability expanded even more with the passage of the Americans with Disabilities Act in 1991, which built the ramps to access the doors opened by Congress.

But there still was—still is—prejudice, and a thinking crip knows that no legislation will ever be written to make discrimination based on mindless suspicion and irrational intolerance illegal.

It all begins with pity, I think. *You are a person with a disability, and therefore you are less than me and need my charity.* And it ends with the assumption that people with disabilities are incapable of controlling their own lives. *You are a person with a disability, and you have no right to decide what is necessary for you to function because you have taken my charity or signed up for my taxpayer-funded program.*

I abhor being pitied, but I also dislike being embarrassed or embarrassing other people. Face to face, those two factors combined mean I am invariably too polite to react angrily when someone imposes their pitiful notion of empathy or compassion upon me.

If someone approaches and says, "It's so sad you're confined to that wheelchair," I'm not going to tell them to mind their own business.

Shit, is my internal response. I admit that. Shit and double shit. But despite my bitter exasperation, I know cynicism—let's call it angry resentment and ill will—is a beast as likely to bite its keeper as anyone else. And so, long ago, in order to keep a fast hold on my sanity, I decided to believe that most people want to do good.

The corollary to that thought is that wisdom comes when we judge cautiously or not at all. I also cling to the sardonic truism that few who pity me because of my disability will be changed by my indignation. Rage will simply reinforce the belief that my spirit is as crippled as my body.

But, dear God, I hate pity. I hate it because once pity is put into words, someone's carefully crafted self-image is going to be fractured. I pity, of course, but because I know pity diminishes and objectifies, I keep it to myself. And I defend my own self-image by refusing to be angered if I sniff pity coming my way.

I learned that riding lesson as I began to think about how humans tend to project their own feelings and reactions onto others. No matter the situation, our egos write a script for a drama in which we play the leading role. Thus, as a crip, I am amused by the black comedy staged when I motor about in public and listen to the silent dialogue—the play will always be staged in the sidelong glances, sometimes moving into stares, the body language, and the soft words directed at minor cast members. Don't stare at the man, honey.

And so I have grown into Gimp, he who has burnt down to the reality of disability. I believe that if you cry for me, most of the tears you shed are for yourself. You can't help it. That's fine. No one would choose disability, not without being tortured, not without being given no choice at all.

And then you will choose disability only because you choose to live.

Until then, go ahead and be glad it's me and not you, at least not yet, at least if you're lucky enough to miss the opportunity. But if you pity me, keep it to yourself. I don't need it, thank you. And I promise to return the favor if misfortune, malevolence, or stupidity sits you down to ride out the rest of your life.

It took me decades of riding lessons to become Gimp, this man who sits below your line of sight and grins at the ironies of life, this man who has only a slippery understanding of who he is and who he appears to be.

That's not to say that I can truly describe either of those people to you. Some days, as the caller said, I'm a fucking loser. It can even happen when someone like me, or someone more active in the disability rights movement reacts to prejudice with the contention that people with disabilities don't need to be cured or fixed.

I find that attitude disingenuous, a blindly cavalier self-assignment of secular semisainthood to people prejudged because of disability.

Of course, disability is "part of human diversity," and people with disabilities should be equal in opportunity even if they are not equal in capacity. But disability is "beautiful" only in spirit, and then only in a few crips.

Some of us are not beautiful at all, neither in body nor in spirit. If disability itself is beautiful, it is not because of its variance from the norm but rather because of its commonality. The beauty of disability is the beauty of being human.

I am a crip, and I cannot be cured, for the disease that sat me down to experience life on wheels is no more. It was a virus smart bomb leaving wry collateral damage. I would be fixed, though, were it possible. I have tasted life above, and I have lived it below, and the view from down here is circumscribed, I will not lie. Sometimes the far horizon, that place toward which I ride, seems a mirage.

23

When I was in my early forties, around 1984, my mother fell ill. For several months, the vibrant woman who carried me into this world shuttled from doctor to doctor. *You've broken your coccyx.* No physician insisted on comprehensive tests. It's *adhesions.* The visits accumulated; appointments were made with new doctors; but what was eventually discovered to be ovarian cancer continued to sap most of her energy as she fought ever-increasing pain.

For more than twenty years, I had relied on my parents for the physical assistance I needed to function in the world. Occasionally my brother stepped in so that they might vacation. I had returned home from the rehabilitation center a near-adult in age but a toddler in my ability to care for my everyday physical needs, and a toddler I remained for two decades, needing help bathing, dressing, using the toilet. A toddler, yes, but a wry, sardonic, overly self-aware one, a strange creature mostly caught up in a sloppy attempt to interpret the world above him from a point of view down below.

During the few weeks after my mother's cancer was discovered and her treatments begun, my father found himself dealing with another strain of the same disease. Alarmed at the stealth of her cancer, my mother urged my father to undergo a thorough physical examination. The doctors found the beginnings of prostate cancer. He chose radiation treatments, drove forty miles alone for the sessions, climbing into his car for the return trip with the beam's target still sketched on his wiry body. The doctors were optimistic, but, as his treatment ended, he became extremely jaundiced. Tests revealed my father had pancreatic cancer.

"Six months to a year," said the doctor.

These words came a few weeks after the same physician told my mother that her cancer had spread to her brain. We fight, we Presleys. In spite of a negative prognosis, my mother chose radiation therapy. Nevertheless, she continued to fade. When she questioned her physician, he responded to her query with a softly phrased measurement of time.

. . . .

She sits in a chair that rocks, reclines, and rotates. She sits still. She is my mother, dressed to meet the day, sweater surrounding shoulders, scarf a vibrant crown. She is bald, wavy dark blond hair burnt away. She is cold, too thin, joints visible, her chin and cheekbones prominent, sallow, all hints of a once robust, even Rubenesque, figure cancer-consumed. Kill her cancer. Soon.

"I don't want to die, Gary," she says, from the border of a country I fear to explore. There is no map I can offer to help her find her way home, none to chart a tranquil journey.

"I know . . ." but I beg—pray—for words to chase the fear from her eyes, fire blue eyes, flickering, hollowing, at her glimpse of the specter slinking.

A day. Another. A nurse. "She's gone," kindly said. Falling into the void, my father and I enter the house. I trail behind him to the bedroom. My mother is dead. Dead because the cancer-beast once more squandered something good. Dead because the cancer-demon moved to her brain. My mother waits for us cancer-dead on her marriage bed—arms covered, eyes closed, face toward heaven. Beneath the cover she holds infinity in the palm of her hand.

I leave my father alone with her.

I have nothing to say. Not even "I know" when my father begins to cry.

. . . .

While my parents had always dedicated themselves to providing the muscle I lacked—lifting me from bed or chair as necessary—my father had rarely volunteered to do the personal chores a quadriplegic needs accomplished—things like trimming toenails, helping with baths, dressing, or the like. Then too, during that period of illness following illness, he had wanted first to devote every particle of his diminishing energy to the care of my mother, as he should have.

That left me, a forty-something dependent person, with two choices. First, I could quit work, open the door to the maze of government bureaucracies, and allow myself to be confined to a nursing home. The word—*confined*—which patronizingly labels an independent wheelchair user begins to fit perfectly when applied to the same person relegated to an institution in which a life disabled is a life regulated by rules and restrictions.

Alternately, I could begin hiring anyone I could find to help me during the morning and evening, primarily with bathing, dressing, and transferring. I intended to fight to preserve as much independence as possible, and so I began calling people I knew who worked or had worked in nursing homes. I understood that seeking help from people experienced with the work of such institutions was probably the simplest way of finding someone who would understand my needs.

Some were reliable. Some were not. Some were careful and attentive. Some wanted only the ten dollars I was willing to pay for the ten minutes of work entailed in helping me transfer. And some left me stranded. Money cannot replace love, nor blood duty.

One night, a year into this ballet of codependence and a few months after my mother was buried, I was forced to call my father to help me transfer from wheelchair to bed, a relatively easy task to accomplish.

Help me secure my hands to the swing bar, grab me under the knees, and then lift and toss, as I direct my launch from chair to bed.

Next, yank off my pants, cover me with the electric blanket, and hand me the supplies I need for the night—urinal within reach, water, aspirin, antacid, telephone.

I knew my father would be angry, and so I waited until far after midnight, hoping against instinct that my attendant was simply late rather than stoned out of her gourd or drunk. All I knew then was that she hadn't shown up to toss me in the sack, and I couldn't tolerate thirty-six hours straight on my ass. Transferring in the evening took only a few minutes. That evening's assistant alternated with another woman, three days one week, four days the next—because no one who doesn't love you will help you every day of every week of every month of every year.

This night it was Trish, the missing person, who was the attendant on the schedule. Gwen assisted me on alternate days. Before I called my father, I called Gwen, but she did not answer her telephone. Trish and Gwen—my legs, my back, the physical links between my desire and my ability to sit up and stand up, to rise up and walk. Trish and Gwen—my independence. Trish and Gwen—to whom I paid a significant portion of my income.

I thought it a bargain.

Trish was a free spirit adorned in peasant blouses, sandals, and the attitude that life was to be enjoyed. That was wardrobe number one. Wardrobe number two was bib overalls and T-shirts. There was no wardrobe three. Trish's husband had left her, and she was mothering a brood of children from that marriage. Trish wrapped up her divorce papers, loaded up her children, and returned to the small town that harbored a business owned by her father and brothers. I had the impression she survived on minimal child support, state aid, and the occasional odd job offering unreported income. Trish lived in a small house on a large lot filled with greenery at the edge of town. Trish loved horses, and she used much of her large lot to corral two geldings.

"That you, Gary?" It was midday Saturday, and Trish was on the telephone.

"Yep. How you doing?"

"Forgot to tell you, sweetie," she said, "Cassie's throwing herself a birthday party. It's gonna be down along the creek near her grandmother's place. Bonfire, barbeque, and beer. You'd be all right, wouldn't you, if I didn't swing by tonight 'til I was on my way home? Say, sometime before midnight?"

"Yeah, no problem. See you then."

But I didn't. Midnight came, and I was tired. Two in the morning came, and I was exhausted.

"Dad, come help me, would you?" I said when I called him. "Trish apparently has forgotten me."

I knew my father, and his nearly unfathomable moodiness, and his sense of duty, and I knew the combination would flare into anger when I explained my predicament. I was right. He was angry when I called him. Angry when I asked for help. Angry when he bounced into my bedroom, angry when he tossed me in bed, and angry when he clicked off the light and left. His touch revealed his emotions if the silence and narrowed eyes had not.

"Thanks, Dad." I called after his retreating form. "I'm sorry I had to bother you." There was no reply, only the shadow of blood obligation met.

Here's an obscene little secret I knew then, had known since I had been stuck in the iron lung, and will know until the day I die: dependency emasculates.

I could have said, *"Why the hell are you mad at me? I'm the one trying to survive by hiring people who don't really care about me. If you're angry with Trish, why are you taking it out on me?"*

But I didn't. I was ashamed. Ashamed of my feeble dependency. Ashamed that I was a man past forty who remained baby-helpless. I accepted his anger as another immutable element of my physical disability. I accepted his anger as reasonable.

Here's another secret: I am a chore.

I will always be a chore, and people don't like chores. People sometimes get angry when they are forced to do chores. How can you love me—or even like me—if I sit here, a helpless lump of obligation? I am such a thing—work, burden, commitment—and I find it perfectly logical that sometimes people will be angry with me.

Maybe it's something akin to a twisted Stockholm syndrome for crips that I've contrived. I have always tried to rationalize why people are sometimes angry when they assist me and why I am fearful of that anger. It is a warped perception, true, and it begins with the knowledge that hostages may come to identify with hostage-takers and leaps to the ugly conclusion that I am a hostage—of my disability, of my need, of someone's willingness to help me. I bend and twist that perception until it nearly breaks, bend it until I begin to believe it was polio that took me hostage. From there, it becomes easy to believe that those who come to rescue me, my caregivers, could be angry with me because I live within the problem.

Actually, I am the problem.

This perception of myself as a chore, a problem, an obligation, descended upon me early, almost as soon as I recognized the extent of my paralysis. Once I recognized that, I jumped head-first into a pool of guilt and began to swim for my life.

Melodramatic? Yes, but look at me. Think of my need for you twice a day, seven days a week, every week of the year. Do that, and then deny I am a problem to be solved, if I pay you, or a duty to be undertaken if you love me. Either way, I am work. Tell me you wouldn't rather have another cup of coffee and linger over the newspaper rather than spend those minutes helping me begin my day.

I require someone to put on my socks, shoes, and pants, and then assist me out of bed each morning. But I cannot let them go about their business even then. They must wait until I need them to help me transfer from a commode chair to my power chair after I have accomplished my toilet. The evening routine spins to a conclusion more quickly, except on those evenings I shower. The sequence then becomes power chair to commode chair, help in undressing, another interlude while I roll into the shower and clean myself, and finally a transfer from commode chair to bed.

Oh, yes. Check my legs and feet before you leave, please. Make sure there are no deep bruises and no toenails becoming ingrown. Bad stuff for a guy like me to get a sore where the circulation is least. I won't call overnight unless something really goes wrong, but keep your telephone where you can hear it, huh?

Count on spending, oh, at least forty-five minutes to an hour a day offering me this care. Seven days a week. Three hundred sixty-five days a year. I spend no days in bed. Never. Bed is retreat. Bed is refuge only when absolutely necessary for sleep. I never linger in bed, not even when ill. In bed, I am wounded and nearly helpless. In bed, I need you. In my wheelchair, I am complete.

There's one caveat. I cannot pay you a fair wage. I am not rich, nor am I even prosperous enough to pay you what you are worth to me. I cannot even love you enough. I am simply a great vacuum, sucking up time and energy you should rightfully be devoting to yourself. I can only promise that I will do my best to be pleasant, perhaps even to entertain you.

As the variety show of attendants entered and exited the stage of my disability, I learned never to stay silent when someone arrived to handle my body. I practiced "instant karma," which meant I remained invariably convivial, concentrating on keeping the mood light, making the situation as palatable as possible for those who were to assist me.

It is ever thus: I choose to be polite in asking for a readjustment when I am not comfortable. "Could you please separate my legs slightly more so that they do not touch in the night? Yes, there. That's much better. You have a good touch. I appreciate it."

And it will always be so: if I am accidentally hurt, if you drop my leg, or yank too abruptly on my shoulders, I will bear down and internalize the pain. I tell myself that any pain you inflict is accidental. I have yet to meet the twisted soul who might choose to hurt me deliberately. Pain is temporary. My need for assistance is permanent.

I learned my lesson early, this necessity to chatter and deflect, to be the good little patient who never complains. The quickest way to find your damaged self at the bottom of the call list in a hospital ward is to be a jerk. Complainers and whiners are dreaded chores. The cheerful and undemanding earn a "Well, we're really not supposed to do that, but . . ." and a quick errand to fetch a magazine or something special from the cafeteria. The foul-mouthed and the never-satisfieds might get lifted, not roughly but abruptly, not out of sadism but in response to the unpleasant environment they are creating. Those dependents who smile, who direct friendly attention to the staff, and who endure the unavoidable discomfort with stoic silence become favorites and benefit from unrushed visits and generous treatment.

It was a game easily played, once I learned the rules. I am an army brat, taught "Yes, sir" and "Thank you, ma'am" from the time I could speak. And, as I became somewhat more sophisticated about the world around me, I began to believe that good manners are also the grease on the wheels of society. Good manners allow us to accomplish what we will. Good manners allow us to substitute words for violence. Good manners make it easy for people to like you.

Of course, congeniality isn't the only way to approach physical dependency. The strong, the powerful, the unafraid will use willpower to dominate and control a situation like mine, but I was too young to be strong when polio ran me down. And as the influence of disability followed me, I remained a teenager, a parent's child, never developing the willpower to influence my own environment because the environment in which I lived was not mine. Thus, once I accepted I had been cooked into quadriplegia, I stopped whining—the quality that earned me bedsores in the hospital—and retreated behind an accepting smile in order to avoid injury, neglect, and abuse. Then after a year or two, I began to believe I had lost control of my life. I could not even defend myself or run away, and so I learned to take the path of least resistance—amiability and passivity.

Given the choice between death—a death I could have earned through willpower—and disability, I bought into disability and chose passive dependence as a bonus. The price seemed high enough, but only later did I come to understand there was also a tax—the emasculation of will.

Things have changed—my acceptance of self, my knowledge of love independent of blood ties—and I have learned to keep the dependence demon at bay most days. I have come to appreciate people as individuals. I try to be openly grateful to everyone who assists me in accomplishing that which my body cannot do for me. "You're so polite," more than one attendant has told me.

Granted, that first choice to be polite, to bite down and swallow my anger, I made because it was in the power of the caregiver to neglect me. And neglecting me would kill me. Now I believe I am polite, and grateful, because I better understand the nature of the transaction.

They are such weak terms—politeness and gratitude—for what I strive to describe as my feelings. I think of what happens between me and the people who care for me—these days my wife and stepsons—as a potent cocktail of reciprocal love, embarrassment, guilt, gratitude, resentment, appreciation, anger, and bemusement, all blended to please the palate and then poured out as a peace offering.

I see the desire to make me comfortable, and I offer a silent toast to the covenant implicit in each movement—the gentle appreciation that she who touches and serves feels both good and bad about helping me, and I, impotent and impatient, feel bad and good about needing her help.

But it's not so simple, this poem I write to those who care for me. To my shame, in spite of my endless rationalizations, I know I will never lose my anger at being dependent upon another person. Anger? No, rage—writhing beneath the pleasant exterior which I strive to show to the world. Rage, running like a stream of molten lava.

God damn it all! Why not just a few more muscles left? Just enough so that I could get in and out of bed by myself. I'm so damn tired of being dependent on people. I want to get in bed by myself, when I want to, not on someone else's schedule. God damn!

Rage, internalized. Rage, unvoiced. Rage once directed at those I hired to assist me but really reflected off them and onto myself for being in a situation where I required help. Incoherent, unjustified, unearned rage; putrid rage, mostly buried, mostly festering into guilt.

Rage then, and now, but never expressed toward those who have helped me because they loved me—never once in the decades I have been a hostage. My mother, primarily, but also my father, my brother, my sister-in-law, my wife, and my stepsons.

Rage at fate—that those who love me must watch while I struggle to swallow all that I cannot, all that I choke on, before finally acknowledging that I have no stomach for it and call for help.

I rarely sensed any resentment from my mother, even in the early days when I was so weak and helpless she would have to roll me onto a bedpan and then wipe waste remnants from my anus. I sensed then the same mother-love that must have flowed from her hands when I was a baby in diapers. I suspect the maternal instinct is drawn out and amplified into love by helplessness. For years I sapped my mother of her time and energy, took away from her all that she might have used for herself, and heard no complaint. I heard, and felt, only genuine, undying concern for my welfare.

Some of the others have approached wearing the cloak of duty. You may choose and discard your friends, but the primitive bonds of blood are difficult to break. I know my father resented the entrance of my disability into his world. What sense did it make to drag himself out of the Depression and learn to prosper through dedication and hard work if my paralysis became his albatross? I know it confirmed his cynicism, his pessimism that doing the right thing might never be enough. I am sorry my brother, his wife, and my stepsons surely have been pulled away from things that they'd rather be doing when asked to assist me.

Now, nearly fifty years in the shadow of dependence, I talk about this ugly sore only with my wife, the woman who chose me after I had been damaged. Only with her do I feel free to speak of the anger in me, anger about me—the anger that has been there in my heart and in my soul; remains there; will always be there.

I say to her, "I don't think about it much anymore, all that bitter anger."

She knows that is one of the few lies I tell her, but she also knows I pray that I will never let the demon harm her.

24

After my mother faded into a coma, lingered a few days, and died, my brother Jon felt the family responsibilities dropped onto his shoulders. But Jon lived ninety miles away, had a daughter in elementary school, a newborn son, and professional obligations as an administrator in his school district.

My father, in the throes of his own illness, seemed to have grown more distant than ever, and so Jon and his family drove down to see us almost every weekend. They would arrive Friday night or early Saturday morning and leave Sunday evening, with Jon's wife, Linda, always bringing food. My father was wasting away, and Linda tried her best to tempt him to eat. Even though every good thing that Linda cooked seemed to do nothing to improve my father's appetite, I could see that Jon, Linda, and their children were able to break through the shell of despair as the pancreatic cancer ate away at him. I am certain he would never have burdened Linda with his fears, and I don't know if he ever opened up to Jon. But alone with me or in the company of those he didn't know, he hid the isolation and terror he felt in response to my mother's death beneath a blanket of silence.

Only once did I see him explode into unnerving tears of loss and despair. During a visit from the Tantons, army friends from decades past, he sat folded into the couch trying to relate the story of my mother's last days and her death. Suddenly, he choked, stopped talking, and began to cry. "I should have gone first. I'm no good without her."

L. M. and Mary Tanton, his friends of thirty years, shuffled in nervous confusion.

Jon's responsibilities were complicated, but he didn't complain. My brother instead worried, becoming frustrated only because my father insisting on driving thirty miles alone in heavy traffic two and three times a week to undergo chemotherapy for his pancreatic cancer. Neither of us said anything, despite our apprehension, when my father refused to sell the horse he treasured—an animal that required daily care—or continued to climb on the tractor to mow, but we both realized the chemotherapy expeditions taxed my father to the depth of his physical resources.

Once home from the eighty-mile round-trip to the specialist in Springfield, my father would retreat to a recliner in front of the television or to his bed to listen to music on the radio. He could eat little. He drank iced tea constantly. He remained silent, twice a day slipping from the house to offer his old quarter horse gelding a pound or two of oats.

Jon had me to worry over also. During the months of my mother's illness and my father's sad diagnosis and treatment, I found myself descending further into a state of mysterious and persistent fatigue, one seemingly beyond measure, one that never relented but progressed toward a state of constant ennui. I was clogged with edema, confused and distant, and sleepy for hours upon hours.

In the face of my mother's downward spiral toward death, in the face of my father's despair and his stoic courage in battling through the storm of chemotherapy, I could not act even as the fatigue and constant sleepiness which had plagued me for years grew worse. I remained frozen in denial. I chose to endure rather than seek out a thorough medical assessment.

What did it matter if I could not remain awake, had no energy, and sat swollen and coughing with edema while cancer consumed my mother and my father prepared to follow her?

Erlyne Pope Presley died in late June 1987, but it took two more months before I gave myself permission to make an appointment for a thorough physical examination. I asked Allie, another of the aides

I'd hired, to drive me. I chose the same clinic, and the same physician, in Springfield where my mother had finally received the treatment she so long needed and failed to receive elsewhere.

I remember now a thorough examination, a quick trip down the block to a hospital for a blood gas test, a return to the physician's office, and finally a hastily arranged, same-day consultation with a pulmonary specialist. Had I been lucid, I would have suspected the hurried sequence of appointments meant I was in serious trouble. It was, after all, a Friday afternoon, a gloriously sunny summer day—a good day for a doctor to head for the lake.

"Be at the hospital Monday," the specialist said. "We need to get you started on a chest shell. Your blood gases are off the chart."

I told my father when we returned home. "Hospital?" he asked. "What do you need to go to the hospital for?"

"Duff sent me to a specialist. The guy said I'm going to need a chest shell."

My father said nothing, but he trusted Dr. Duff, the physician who had cared so compassionately for my mother and was now offering him the best support possible in a bad situation.

I knew then—or, at least I understood, given the fragile courage with which I approached my disability in its early stages, a courage that allowed me to endure but not to act—that it was my father's will which had driven me off the rocking bed and away from the clutches of the respiratory pneumatic belt. I suppose my father, like me, clung to the belief that once free of mechanical respiratory assistance I would remain free for the rest of my days. Neither of us had heard of post-polio syndrome.

I called my brother and relayed the word. "I'll be down to drive you," Jon said. It was summer. School wasn't in session.

I bought pajamas, or rather Linda bought some for me. I had slept nude at home, draping myself with a beach towel for privacy during transfer and while being dressed.

Blue pajamas, a book, an electric razor, a toothbrush, all in a brown satchel on my lap. I remember watching idly, sleepily, as a clerk flipped paper and asked for my signature.

And then I was assigned a room, and I was lifted into a hospital bed. *Strange*, I thought. *I have lived twenty-seven years in a wheelchair, but not a day in a hospital since 1960.*

Then nothing. A void. Black oblivion.

I entered the hospital on a sunny Monday afternoon in August 1987. Today, I recall the room, a nurse, and the fuzzy knowledge of something off-kilter and imprecise about where I found myself. I think I approached the stay with anticipation rather than dread. I believed the chest shell would help me. I wanted to feel better. I felt only slightly nervous about the unfamiliar surroundings.

But the next three or four days are empty. Empty of sensations, self-awareness, and even dreams.

"Are you okay?" a nurse asks shortly after Jon and my father leave. I am in a hospital bed. She reaches for my wrist, and I rest my head on the pillow.

I try to look at her closely. Scrubs, solid-colored pants, patterned top. Brunette, wavy hair cascading below her ears. Thirties, forties. Twenty pounds overweight for her height by Hollywood standards, but proportionately feminine, a lushly attractive woman.

"You sure?" She touches my head.

"Huh? Oh, yeah, I'm okay," I reply. She stares intently, turns, and I watch her merge into the hallway traffic. I like women.

Then, limbo. No pain. No dreams. No bright lights. No angels. A quick descent into nothingness.

The biological engine that drives me through this world sputters and stops. Experts are called. I am revived. The engine stops once more. Again, experts—anesthesiologists, wizards wielding magic intubations. Four times in all. I remember nothing.

So different, those days, from that great whirlwind of illness when polio raged through my life in 1959.

Then: *I am ill; therefore, I am.* Alive. In pain. In confusion. In people, moving, talking. Noise. Light.

Now, no burning mad dreams or fractured delusions. No awareness of my plight. Oblivion.

Post-polio syndrome arrived quietly, moving toward me sneakily, first appearing, it seems, when I didn't fully recover from a horrendous bout of the flu in 1979. I had not recognized post-polio syndrome because it was masquerading as the normal evolution of aging. Nevertheless, it ate away at my life. I had been for two years, or three, or four, a candle burning, then flickering. Now the flame sputtered, shedding no light in the void of those lost days in August.

No dreams, no bizarre visions, no mirages—only an absence of self, an abyss into which I entered without falling or floating.

I am ill; therefore, I am not.

Post-polio syndrome is a phantom disease to some in the medical field, one to be cured with placebos and counseling.

"You're paralyzed," begins the dismissal. "People in wheelchairs are going to age differently than normal people. You're going to have more aches, pains, and fatigue."

Yes, true. True also that many in the medical profession were slow to understand that, while disability is not necessarily a disease, diseases strike people with disabilities—that something can come from the paralysis engendered by polio rather than be caused by it.

I hate hypochondria, and the bastard child of that intolerant emotion is my belief that some people with disabilities are in essence hypochondriacs. Why should it be otherwise if a person chooses to become their disability?

The corollary to that ugly prejudice is that I believe the first diagnosis that often pops into a physician's mind when presented with a person with a disability is hypochondria. Too often, in the physician's mind a person with a disability is already sick, already in need, already has something wrong.

I admit that assumption reeks with ignorance and cynicism, but, for years uncounted, I know society treated disability as illness, and so my attitude toward hypochondria certainly was a protective reaction. I know too many people with disabilities swallowed legitimate health complaints in order not to be perceived as wimpy, whining invalids. And there, in that foolish blanket reaction to the idea that illness is weakness, I find the attitude that became the impetus for my eight-year struggle with post-polio syndrome, a struggle I eventually and inevitably lost.

There are other reasons, of course, that aggravated my inability to understand that I was descending toward collapse. For example, there is no single test that can identify post-polio syndrome. Looking back on those years, I can only suggest the syndrome is as real as the pain, the increasing weakness, and the intermittent collapses from fatigue. Some research I've since read indicates that post-polio syndrome apparently occurs more often in males than females. It generally strikes decades after the onset of the original disease. And it focuses mostly in those who came away with a significant degree of paralysis after the bout with the virus.

Interestingly, post-polio syndrome began showing up in the 1970s. Why then and not earlier? Primarily, I think, because evolving medical care and drugs had sustained those caught up in the epidemics of the 1940s and 1950s into middle age and older.

Researchers who identify post-polio syndrome as a complication of the original disease suggest it most likely strikes those who were forced to compensate for a wide-ranging degree of diminished muscle capacity. That leaves the remaining muscles (and the nerve pathways driving them) subject to early deterioration because of long-term overwork. Often, the catalyst is another debilitating illness—in my case, I think, that severe flu infection, during which I ran a temperature of a hundred and four degrees for nearly a week.

Why did it take me too many years to understand that something was terribly wrong? I can only tell you I fought it—fought it as I battled all the other constraints imposed by my paralysis—refusing to give in, ignorant and disbelieving in this strange malady's power to kill. I fought it, misinformed and improperly treated after inept diagnoses. I fought it, perceived by doctors as doomed simply because I used a wheelchair. I fought it, growing more confused and weakened, until I slipped into the void on that Monday afternoon in a room at St. John's Regional Health Center.

Looking back, I can see it was only a year or two following that nasty flu attack that I began to feel weak and unfocused, sleeping restlessly and awakening without energy. I began to complain to the very few people I trusted, but not to my father, who clung to the belief that unless the bleeding could not be stopped or a limb was misaligned a man had an obligation to soldier on. I agreed, silently thinking I was becoming what I liked least—a hypochondriac.

Then, a year or two before my mother's illness was discovered, I finally gave in, and I brought up my ever-growing weakness and unrelenting fatigue to one of the general practitioners who had seen me through minor illnesses and injuries in the decades following my paralysis.

Dr. Wallace was then three or four decades into his practice, a busy small-town doctor with a penchant for hopping into his twin-engine airplane and flying off to satisfy his interest in golf outings and offshore yachting.

Dr. Wallace, without malice but without curiosity, undertook every wrong thing medically possible after I approached him with my complaints. Is it possible that he didn't expect me—or anyone—to be alive, let alone be healthy enough to keep living, after more than twenty years in a wheelchair? Then there is this. If you act like something is killing you, I suppose the obvious response is for someone to treat you as if you're dying.

Dr. Wallace listened to my chest and began treating me for heart failure. Repeated visits resulted in prescriptions for different kinds of diuretics. Nothing worked. I still had severe fluid retention. I still woke each morning feeling as if I hadn't slept at all. I began to weaken further. Pain was constant. Palatable pain. Worse, I began to nod off regularly during the day, even at work, even in the middle of an ongoing conversation.

More visits to Dr. Wallace. Golden hair. Slim, compact body. Bright harried eyes of a man making early morning hospital rounds and then seeing fifty patients a day to support a large family and extravagant avocations. "How's the diuretic doing with the edema?" he asked.

"It's making me pee. That's about all I can say," I replied.

More prescriptions.

Me, too dazed to object. Too afraid to give into the idea that I was ill and nothing, no one was helping.

Too addled, it's true, to look into the doctor's clear blue eyes and read, "*Ah, shit, what a mess. People in wheelchairs aren't meant to live a normal lifespan. This guy had twenty years after bulbar and lumbar polio, and now he's suffering.*"

The muscles I had used the hardest, used without respite, over the decades following polio were those muscles I used to breathe, and so what had been inordinate fatigue and pain and restless sleep soon began to spiral down into respiratory insufficiency.

The pattern of drifting off at random moments moved from evenings to any hour of the day. I fell asleep while eating, while brushing my teeth—once even losing consciousness while using my urinal, awakened only as the stainless steel jar clattered and splashed on the tile floor of my bathroom. Even choosing to nap for an hour or so while sitting in the wheelchair didn't alleviate the constant sleepiness. Nothing helped, and the edema creeping from my feet to my ankles to my calves seemed to chart my descent toward collapse.

Toward the end, as my mother lingered in a coma in her bedroom, I eventually became so tired and drained that even after a long night's sleep I would head directly toward a small respirator—a Zephyr by name, a machine that discharged a constant stream of air at about thirty pounds of pressure—I had kept as a safety device for years. The little Zephyr had been sent home with me from the rehabilitation center by the March of Dimes almost three decades previously. Its purpose was to exercise my lungs, to inflate them with more air than I could draw in naturally, to stretch them. In emergencies, I could use it to inhale enough air to generate a cough.

Now the Zephyr became a touchstone, the magic wind that kept me alive as I raced toward eventual collapse.

I kept the Zephyr in my bathroom. I began the morning by rubbing the sleep from my eyes, splashing water on my face, and then reaching for the precious, restful flow of air available at the flick of a switch. I would clasp the feeder tip between my teeth, shaving, sitting over the stool, surviving. Air without the expenditure of energy. Sweet air, with the faint taste of metal and rubber.

Thus, my "coughing machine" became a "resting machine." But the resting machine only delayed the day I was finally forced to recognize that I wasn't breathing correctly while asleep, that a combination of residual viral damage and neuromuscular weakness was pushing me steadily toward the void.

Even with the Zephyr adding an hour or two of true rest every day, I still had severe fluid retention. I still woke each morning feeling as if I hadn't slept at all. I still didn't have sufficient energy to make it through my nine-hour workday. I began falling asleep at my desk. Toward the end of my fight with post-polio syndrome, I remember working on computer records while the agency owner escorted one of the company adjusters to the front door. I watched them through my office window looking into the reception area of the insurance agency. They paused. Suddenly I heard, "What's wrong with Gary?"

My head snapped up, my neck weak and wobbly as a noodle. I had come awake to the sound of my name.

"I don't know," my boss said, a man who was ignoring his deteriorating hearing like I was ignoring post-polio syndrome. He carried on his conversations at twice the volume necessary. Although he didn't intend so, his voice carried into my office. "I've been trying to get him to see another doctor, but he won't do it."

My neck wobbles. My eyes close. I snap them open. I grasp the control of my wheelchair and move about the office to keep awake. I am tired once again. I stop and rest my head against my hand. What's he saying? My eyelids drift down, and I open them by biting the inside of my lip.

I had reached the stage where my life became *Move or fall asleep.* Such an odd thing, this gently suffocating killer, this post-polio-driven sleep apnea, this inability to ventilate correctly while asleep—so immutable that the power of will can fail and the power of ignorance can kill.

But still tenacious in my refusal to be perceived as one more weakling in a wheelchair, I ignored the effects of the apnea. I ignored the pain, fatigue, and weakness.

Dropping off while eating, in mid-chew, and awakening with a gag; falling toward the bathroom mirror while brushing my teeth; drifting into a head-bob while words tumbled from a customer's mouth—I remember each one, the long days of confusion and oppression, and I am sorry I allowed passivity—ignorance—to almost kill me.

It is the absence of dreams I think about most when I recall the hole in my life. I suppose I was sick nearly to death, living somewhere beyond coherent thought, somewhere even my subconscious could not reach me, a place beyond dreams. No dreams as I struggled through those last months of my mother's illness. No dreams as I fretted about my father's fatal reckoning.

And no dreams as I drifted off after the nurse left my hospital bedside.

Where did I go in those days? How did I go?

I did not linger in the confusion of Alzheimer's, where demons eat memory. Nor did I travel to the island of the brain-injured, that silent place hidden from watchers by tubes and beeping machinery.

It frightens me to think I drifted down through months of confusion to land in a hospital bed where I became a thing, a clot of meat on a slab, brain sufficient only to lurk at lizard level, there to engineer survival.

I was Gary no more, not for those lost days, not the me of sardonic wit covering a suit of self-awareness stitched together from self-pity, stubbornness, and sad frustration. I was probed and prodded, tossed and turned, and moved from bed to bed and room to room. Tubes were sent up into my bladder and down into my throat. Lungs were pumped full of air and emptied. Fluids were inserted and drained. All this without id or ego, heart beating perversely. Body alive—a minuscule organism in a universe of one hundred billion times one hundred billion stars. Body alive—a nanoscopic collection of atoms sustained by little engines of care: a respirator, a catheter, a bottle of fluids, and a needle.

Days gone. A memory. Thursday? My brother and father stand on each side of a bed, behind them a backdrop of machines, lights flashing in rhythm with clicks and beeps.

"Can you hear me?" my brother asks. "Are you waking up?" Jon squeezes my arm.

I cannot speak. There is a tube crunched down my throat to feed me air.

"You're on a respirator," Jon says. "You kept falling asleep, and then your breathing would decrease, nearly stop. No one could wake you. They've had to resuscitate you. Four times. You're in the ICU."

I nod, and then I drift off again, not into the void this time, but rather into fits of sharp pain and restless discomfort, gagging on the ventilator tube, legs rigid and cramping.

Jon tells me that each time the anesthetist came to revive me I was given morphine.

"I told them it would only make your breathing worse," he says. "But they needed it to get the tube down your throat."

My father nods. He is wrapped around his own cancer. He has given control of my treatment over to Jon.

I trust Jon.

The morphine was meant to keep me from fighting against intubation. But my body was shutting down because of respiratory insufficiency, and the morphine exacerbated the problem.

During the battle, Dr. Heinz, the pulmonary specialist who had admitted me, tried a chest shell, the same sort of device I used when transitioning out of the iron lung nearly three decades previously. With the shell, I revived slightly but only briefly, and then, once again, my body shut down. But now, dangling at the end of life's tether, the sustained use of a positive pressure respirator had halted my respiratory collapse and began to restore my blood gases and rid my blood of killing carbon monoxide.

Time is irrelevant in an intensive care unit. I do not know when Dr. Heinz made his first visit to explain my predicament.

"The only alternative is a tracheotomy," he concluded, "after which you will need to use a respirator." Two nurses flanked him. My father and brother stood at the bedside.

I shook my head, signaling no. I could not speak because the respirator tube remained down my throat. My father grimaced in anger, his belief that my inclination was always to make the wrong choice verified. My brother said nothing.

"Without it, you'll die," Heinz said. He had thick dark hair and dark eyes, which were somberly highlighted against his white lab jacket.

I shook my head once more and mimed the act of writing with paper and pen. The male nurse lifted a clipboard and flipped a sheet of paper over before handing the board to me.

Consult? I wrote.

"Sure," Heinz replied after glancing at the paper. "Who?"

The name came quickly. I recalled the story in a magazine devoted to disability interests. I reached for the clipboard again. I wrote, *Dr. Oscar Schwartz. Post-polio expert. St. Mary's Hospital. St. Louis, Missouri.*

It was Schwartz who explained to Dr. Heinz the nature of neuro-muscular-induced sleep apnea. It was Schwartz who outlined a program of noninvasive mechanical respiration—a small, portable respirator feeding a nasal mask. Schwartz arranged for one of the devices to be delivered to the hospital, brought by a respiratory therapist who specialized in noninvasive ventilation. That technician would help the doctor guide my adaptation to the unit. It was Schwartz who kept me alive and set me on the road to good health.

Two days later, I left the ICU for a regular hospital room. Five days after that I moved back home to watch my father die of pancreatic cancer.

. . . .

My brother sits in an armchair, his back to the north window of the hospital. One day. Another. A third. Each day I watch the spare clouds lurking behind sparkling glass as I finesse my way—once, twice, again, once more—along the narrow space separating hospital beds from the wall. One bed is empty. Waiting. The other cradles my father, racing toward sunset.

One breath. Ragged. Flutter. Silence. Space. Another breath. Rattle. Jaw flap-heave.

Another day. Twenty-three before. Dry-burnt grass. Heat. My father, erect and bone-thin. Rock-hard. Cane-pinned to earth. Kneeling, above my mother's stone, white roses in hand. A "sentinel of the grave who counts us all."

Another breath calls me back from grave-memory. Broken. Jagged. Silence-space. Reaching further toward eternity each minute, hour, day.

Jon stands. "We best go." I nod.

Another breath. Flutters. Silence. Space. Words. Clear.

"This is the hardest part," my father says. Eyes closed. Legs move. Another step toward the precipice in the fading light.

"I know . . ." I say. At last. Empty. Alone.

25

"Don't wear that jacket," one of my cousins said. "Too hot out here."

It was the bright hot last day of July 1988, and we had arrived at Springfield National Cemetery. I'd exited my van, and Linda handed me my suit jacket. We were ready to bury my father in the grave he would share with my mother, who had died one year and one month previously. Family and friends—twenty, thirty, forty—lingered near a tent covering the coffin. The grave was fifty yards east, settled in the shade of a pavilion honoring the dead from the bloody Civil War battle at Wilson's Creek.

I watched a military honor guard contingent from Fort Leonard Wood begin to gather. A squad would render honors, escort the coffin, fire a twenty-one-gun volley, and present a flag. None knew my father. They were simply symbols of his service, symbols I doubt he would have wanted. He joined the Retired Officers Association only to buy discounted supplementary health insurance, and he showed no interest in the American Legion or the Veterans of Foreign Wars. The presence of the honor guard was a decision left to Jon and me. We were proud that our father had given more than twenty years in service to his country.

Our family—my father's nieces and nephews so close in age to be almost his contemporaries, Jon and his family, and me—sweated under the temporary canvas awning. Tim McManus, my friend from high school, the friend who lifted me into his car and drove me to church for several months when I first returned home from the rehabilitation center, the friend who spent dozens of years preaching in the slums of Managua, Nicaragua, before the Sandinista National Liberation Front sent him home to Missouri, offered a few words about the man who was an acquaintance rather than a friend or a parishioner.

Then the honor guard assembled in the hundred-degree heat. I noticed they were in dark Class A uniforms. "I wonder why they're wearing winter greens," I said to my brother. He didn't reply. And the volleys began—seven M16s, a rifle first used by the U.S. Army ten years after my father retired—three volleys. Flat, sharp cracks. Jon's daughter and son, a grade-schooler and a toddler, flinched but did not cry.

Other soldiers removed the flag from the coffin—the coffin we chose because it was identical to the one my father selected for my mother—and a young lieutenant handed me the flag.

I was left to carry it to the house where I now would live alone, my parents' home, one of the three places I have lived with them since being freed from the iron lung, through the isolation of my twenties, after my release into the world during my thirties, and now, in sickness and in health, in my forties. One thing has changed. I am divorced from the belief that I will always be dependent upon—as I always have been—family for care.

Upon the death of my father, Jon and I decided to sell the house and the twenty acres surrounding it. However, until the apartment I would rent was modified for wheelchair accessibility, I would live in my parents' house alone, relying on Trish to fetch me home from work each day and assist me into bed. I would be alone throughout the night, on my back, in my bed, holding hard to the box containing my fears of claustrophobia, holding hard to keep from panicking and then screaming witlessly into the empty night. Alone three miles from town with only a telephone available to call for help, waiting for Allie, my morning shift attendant, to arrive at six the next morning to dress me, lift me from the bed, and drive me to work.

"Who's going to take care of you now?" asked Eileen, my employer's wife. We were in the hallway outside the room where my father was waiting to die. She and her husband, Richard, the insurance agent for whom I had worked for more than a decade, had come to see him one last time.

"No one. I'm staying by myself. Except for Allie and Trish coming to help me transfer."

"That's crazy," she said. Richard nodded his head in agreement. "You need to go into the nursing center," she continued.

"Can't afford it," I said. That was only partly true. I could have burnt through every dollar in my accounts paying for a few months of nursing-home care, after which I could have quit work altogether, signed up for aid, and turned my life over to government bureaucracies and the nursing-home industry. But I knew if I entered a nursing center—the place most people assumed was a logical refuge for a crip, incapable of getting in or out of bed, let alone wiping their own ass—I would never leave. And I would die sooner rather than later, a process I was certain would begin the minute I turned management of my condition over to a system where no single person felt as responsible for my welfare as I did.

"Ah, don't worry," I said. "The independent living apartment will be ready soon." That seemed to deflect some of Eileen and Richard's frustration, but I knew they probably thought that choice inappropriate as well.

I actually thought I would be in no more peril in my parents' suburban house than I would be in the apartment in town. In both places, I would be alone throughout the night, every night. I might wake up to fire, or my respirator might fail, or . . . who knows? The dark imaginings of people who thought me foolish were only murmurs in the face of the terrors screaming in my ear. I was afraid, but I was more afraid of giving up, retreating to a nursing home. I understood life could play funny tricks when a person was in bed and unable to move. But I ignored my fears and rationalized that the only difference when I moved to town would be that help was stationed two blocks away rather than three miles away. Of course, it would also mean that there in the apartment I would be relying on people with whom I had no extended relationship.

I liked the apartment—which was more like a very small house—when I inspected it during the negotiation of our agreement. The sturdy brick structure had a single door that opened into a foyer. I noticed a bathroom equipped with a roll-in shower directly opposite the entrance. To the right was a bedroom, sixteen by twenty feet, and to the left, a sitting room and kitchenette of the same dimensions. The little building was located on the five-acre estate of the owner of the nursing center. I expect the original owner of the estate, proprietors of an area lumber company, had built it as mother-in-law quarters or as a guest cottage. For my purposes, the little house was private, secure, and, best of all, bore no resemblance to anything institutional.

This new adventure—which was scheduled to cost me close to a thousand dollars a month—was another reminder of how expensive an avocation being a crip can be. From the day I realized I would ride out the rest of my life on my fanny, I began to learn the single thing that I lacked that would make my life better was money, and a lot of it. Had I inherited massive amounts from my parents, had I invested in Wal-Mart stock when Sam had only a few dozen stores, had I been struck by the lightning of a winning lottery ticket, I could have built a dwelling configured for a wheelchair user and hired full-time, round-the-clock personal care attendants.

For a crip, the root of all independence, which is good rather than evil, is money.

I had paid Trish and Allie three hundred dollars a month each for less than an hour's worth of work a day on average. Nevertheless, I think they chose to assist me because they found satisfaction in providing care for another person. Both were natural caregivers, and the one night that Trish had forgotten me proved to be the only time she put me in jeopardy.

After I moved to the small apartment on the grounds of the nursing home, I began to understand what I had lost when I gave up attendants who seemed to have some emotional investment in my welfare. The nursing home attendants that initially arrived to help me were not volunteers. They were assigned to the task. They were ordered to leave the facility, drive or walk the two short blocks to my apartment, and, once there, follow my instructions. Some didn't mind, taking the trip as an opportunity to get fresh air and escape supervision. Some seemed fearful of me. And some were the wrong people for the job.

I had never visited a nursing center, but, as I met the variety of people sent to assist me, I began to believe that many of the elderly relegated to the wrong sort of warehouse for the incapable could easily be neglected or even bullied if an attendant chose to do so. When I encountered that sort—admittedly only one or two in the years I contracted for care with the center—I confronted them as a person who intended to direct how he was helped. Once outside the boundaries of people who cared about my everyday welfare—parents, family, and attendants-turned-friends—I fast became the sort to speak out, to get angry when I perceived I was being handled by someone who obviously resented being sent to aid me.

"Damn! Careful!" The pain burnt through my toe, across and around my ankle, and up my calf. "I think you caught a toenail on the sock."

"No, I didn't." It was morning, and there was a woman dressing me, slipping on my shoes and socks and pulling my pants to my knees before helping me into the commode chair. It was the first time she had been sent to assist me. Once I was up, she would then return to the center. I would telephone when finished with the bathroom, and another person would come to transfer me into my power wheelchair.

Thin yet curvy, in her thirties, with dark hair pulled together and flowing down her back, the aide evidently hadn't wanted the assignment—or at least her demeanor seemed to make that clear. She wouldn't look at me. She hadn't looked at me when she opened the door and called, "I'm from the center." She hadn't looked at me when I explained what I needed.

"How long have you worked for ANC?" I asked after she entered my bedroom. "First time I remember you coming over." Normally, the supervisor would send someone new with a person who had assisted me previously.

"A couple of months," the dark-haired woman replied. "They're running short this morning. Told me I had to come over here."

The *had to* was the telling comment. *Had to* meant my foot would be matted with blood from a ripped-off toenail when the attendant undressed me that night.

"What happened here?" Jim asked. "Your foot's a mess."

"I don't know. I can't see that far without my glasses. I know it hurt like hell when the woman they sent over this morning put on my support socks."

"She ripped off your damn toenail. Off your little toe. Shit. That ain't good," Jim said. He moved to the bathroom, found some hydrogen peroxide, and began to clean my foot.

After he left, I called and left a message for the nursing supervisor. I didn't want that woman sent over again.

Initially, five or six different people might show up during any week, but, by the first winter after I moved into the apartment, my aides had dwindled to a group of regulars. The occupational therapist technician at the center became my weekday morning regular. Short, square, and swift, Jeannie would bang through the door and have me out of bed within minutes.

At night, it was usually a man, the night supervisor at the center being reluctant to send a woman along the deserted street in the dark. No doubt a few of the female aides were also reluctant to visit the apartment, help a man into his bed, and there undress him. Sometimes at night the women came in pairs, as if they believed I had found a television evangelist who sent a miracle down the cable, and I would be standing by the door ready to demand sex from the first woman who crossed the threshold.

Despite my conscientious attention to avoid any touch, any word that might be considered improper, only a few women were willing to come alone. One was a young mother of two named Belinda Baldwin. "Like the piano," she replied when I asked her name. I always asked names and used them. Living disabled in this world requires political skills of the first order.

The first evening she arrived to help, she had accompanied one of the older women. "Do you know how to use a socket wrench?" I asked with a smile. I had noticed part of the assembly of my shower chair was loose, and I wanted it tightened before I transferred to take a shower.

"Sure," she replied. "I helped my father all the time when I was growing up."

"Well, there's a set in the lower left drawer of my desk. Get it, and I'll show you how this thing goes back together."

That's when I asked her name. I didn't have any conception that in four years it would be Presley.

26

When Belinda and I met, she was approaching her twenty-seventh birthday, two semesters short of completing a college degree in biology. Her higher education spanned a decade because she had to work as a nurse's aide to finance her schooling and pay for daycare for her two sons. During that winter of 1989, Belinda was juggling family demands, scholastic choices, minimal income, and guilt evolving into apprehension over the collapse of a marriage to a man—a boy, really—who neither loved nor appreciated her, whose neglect and indifference sometimes reverted to passive-aggressive obstruction and emotional abuse.

As our acquaintance grew, Belinda would sometimes stop by the apartment on her way to begin her three-to-eleven shift. We became friends, two people with a constant curiosity about the world around us and our place in it. We talked about my work and hers, her opportunities to go to graduate school, and her dreams. Neither one of us realized at first that her dreams were to include me.

Cynics say romance is a fiction, perhaps even a willful blindness overlooking long-term self-interest and focusing on short-term self-gratification. I think love is a mystery, an enigma, a puzzling Gordian knot entwining two spirits. I cannot say why my mother loved my father. I cannot tell you why my brother married his wife. And I have never been able to resolve myself to the reality of what happened between Belinda and me, how we were able to ignore the demands my paralysis would make on a wife, how we chose intimacy and companionship over isolation, how we chose without regret to sacrifice for one another.

I only know it happened quickly, and it took a relatively long time, and it will last forever.

We met in late 1988, with Belinda married. By May 1989, Belinda had graduated with a B.S. in biology and gained admittance to an accelerated Ph.D. program at Texas A&M University. Then her husband refused to leave Missouri, even though he had only a routine line job in a local factory and no ambition to improve. To save her marriage—and because she could not support her two young boys on the stipend offered by the university—she turned down the Ph.D. program and instead enrolled in a local university to seek a master's in microbiology and immunology, a field she found fascinating. A month later, July 1989, her husband bought a new car, drove over to the nursing center where she was working full-time during her summer vacation, and announced that he was leaving her and filing for divorce.

That left Belinda with two children, a job slightly above minimum wage, and a reluctance to turn to her family because she didn't want to hear, "You made your bed, now lie in it."

That bed was moved to a public housing apartment in the town where I lived, which was a short commute to Springfield, where her university was located. Toward the end of the summer before her classes got underway, I began to assist her with Christopher and Matthew, her two boys, providing after-school childcare while she ran errands or going with her when she took them to the zoo or for other outings.

As our time together increased, she began to teach me things smart men learn early in a courtship. Three months after her divorce, we were driving toward Springfield in my van. "I need a second opinion on what a professional woman should wear," she had told me when she asked me to come along. The master's program allowed her a chance to supplement her income by working as a graduate teaching assistant, and she wanted to look the part.

"One of these days, I'm going to find one of those and rebuild it," she said as we approached the edge of Springfield. She was pointing to a restored early model VW Beetle in the adjacent lane. I was only half listening, drifting along with my own thoughts, perhaps wondering why there seemed to be a connection between me and this woman twenty years my junior.

"If wishes were horses, beggars would ride," I said, without thinking.

"What a mean thing to say," she snapped, turning her head away.

I twisted forward to look at her. She was driving. My power wheelchair was locked in the metal bracing located behind the front seat. I didn't understand what I'd done by voicing the ancient aphorism.

"People have a right to dream," she said.

I thought about her reaction and apologized by buying lunch. Belinda bought dresses, asking my opinion as she tried on each one. She liked floral prints. I liked a navy blue one with white polka dots.

When we returned to my apartment, she sat on my couch with her legs tucked under her, looking away from me, out the window at the cedar trees along the driveway. I told her, again, that I hadn't meant to hurt her feelings.

"It's all right," she replied. "I shouldn't be so sensitive."

I watched her, saying nothing. I could see despair in the way she held her shoulders.

"Would you think me a slut if . . . if I told you something," she paused, ". . . no, asked you something?"

"No, I don't think so . . ." I didn't understand. "Slut . . ." it wasn't the sort of word I expected from her. She seemed shy around her coworkers, although she became more open and outgoing when we were alone and talking about things other than my need to be transferred from wheelchair to bed or shower chair.

"Would you . . . would it be . . .? Could you please just hold me?" she asked. "It's been . . . years since anyone has held me without wanting something."

I simply nodded my head.

Belinda raised herself from the couch and crossed the two or three steps between us. I opened my arms, and she sat in my lap and rested her head on my shoulder. There was no sound, no words between us, but I soon felt her tears dampen my shirt.

"Bed is the poor man's opera," says an Italian proverb. Belinda, the fire of Sicily in her paternal bloodline, had been married, in name if not in practice, but she'd never had a lover. No one had taught her to sing.

It is probably not important for me to identify the time when friendship flowered into passion, or the day when hugs of support changed to affectionate caresses or the night when the tears ended with kisses. I only remember the gift, the magic, the seamless transition from what I could never imagine into what I will treasure until my last breath, and beyond.

Dark bedroom, ethereal glow of far away streetlights shadowing the windows, the sweet, hot touch of skin to skin, the fears, reassurances, and promises whispered.

Friends first, lovers next—hearts beating in rhythm, then the playful song of laughing intimacy, as we learned to dance to life's subtle music, never alone.

And so it may have been a year after her divorce when Belinda and I began to integrate our couplehood into her family. Whether by calculation or instinct, I can't tell you, Belinda resolved to show them, and perhaps me, that what we were together—a blending of male and female, of love and support, of need and fulfillment—bound us in a way that incorporated my disability as an element of the union.

We also began to make short trips together, and Belinda learned my disability was supported by a framework of logistics. I grew impatient, petulant, confused, and she pulled back, attempting to determine how much my disability would cost her. We learned that intimacy demanded we deflect our anger and frustrations away from each other's vulnerabilities. I learned gentleness. She learned she could bear part of my weight. And we both learned that sorrow shared is a burden lightened.

Another year passed, and we were apart less, and together more.

She said, "We're going to get married." I could not agree. Her father disapproved of her passion for our union, of her refusal to move out of my orbit.

"I've told her to see other people," I said to him, "but she refuses."

"She's like her mother," he replied. "She wants someone to take care of. She needs to be needed." The disapproval was evident, as though he were blind to the care, the old-world submissiveness, Belinda's mother offered—lavished upon—him.

I knew that might be so—that Belinda might see in me a thing to nurture, a place to sacrifice, an altar on which to offer love. I could feel it in Belinda's touch. But I could also feel something else in her touch—the heat between a female and her mate.

I cannot explain why we didn't marry for three years. Seasons drifted from one into another. It became routine when we were together for her to help with my transfers before she drove home to her apartment. "Call the center. Tell them I'll help you into bed," she'd say.

One afternoon she showed me a man's wedding ring, a wide band with oak leaves inlaid into its surface. "I had it made," she said, "a few days after you told me you would be the best friend I'd ever have. See if it fits."

"It's not right," I replied. "We can't marry. You have no business pulling my burdens into your life."

"It's my choice," Belinda said. "Besides, I need you. I know that. I am sure. I just can't give you the words that explain the reasons."

"You need to find someone your age, Belinda," I told her. "You don't need to be saddled with a crip."

Her only worry was that I would want a woman who might give me children. "I can't have any more kids, you know," she said. "Not since I've had a hysterectomy."

Then Belinda secured a three-week educational sabbatical in Canberra, Australia, at the Commonwealth Scientific and Industrial Research Organization. The days apart only further convinced her that she wanted to be married to me. She returned directly from the airport and closed the door to my apartment behind her.

"I don't care about the chair. I don't care how old you are. I don't care about anything—just marry me and give me five years. Then I can make it."

"No, baby," I replied. "You don't want to tie yourself to me. It's not right."

I had loved women all my life—cherished them, or at least cherished the image and character of Woman I had conceived from the females around me. I had worked with women. I had had women as friends. But I had never really dated seriously or had a deep and loving relationship with a woman.

I simply never had the courage to imagine resigning from the place I felt I occupied in the world—a brother in the Monastery of Cripdom—and entering into life as a married man.

A married man carries his bride over a threshold; he changes the oil in her car and mows the lawn; he goes to work every morning and then takes his family camping and water-skiing on the weekends. A married man does not need help getting out of bed and dressing every morning; he does not revert to part-time work at age forty-five because he must husband his energy; he does not seek an early bedtime to avoid overexertion and then reach for a CPAP respirator because his breathing shuts down at night.

There were unattached women in my life before Belinda. Susan, a Rubenesque schoolteacher. Maggie, a girl I knew in high school who sometimes showed up to chat and borrow books. Carrie, the unmarried daughter of an acquaintance, a woman nearly my age, who may have preferred nephews to children and busyness to friendship. I had lived two decades into my disability as a single man, clinging discontentedly to my fantasies, blind to any vision of myself as a lover and husband. Whenever any single woman entered my orbit, I immediately invested myself in the idea that an overture on my part would result in rejection. I knew I would be rejected. I lacked the courage to face it.

I didn't understand why it was different with Belinda. "What do you want with me anyway?" I asked her regularly.

"I like older men," she replied. "Don't you think Sean Connery is sexy? How about the guy who plays Jean-Luc Picard on television? You remind me of them, especially with your hair short."

"But what do you think when you see the wheelchair?"

"I don't see it, really," she replied.

"You're a strange girl."

Am I married because Belinda saw what she wanted, what she needed, in me? I think so. She wanted loyalty, support even when she failed, and the completeness of a man perceiving her as a soul who might make his own spirit whole rather than as a vessel for his passions, as a housemate willing to cook and clean, and as a source of income to help support his hobbies.

Was I not married before I met Belinda because I didn't trust myself or a woman's perception of me? I think so. Even now I find it odd. I always liked women. My father, albeit something of a male chauvinist who thought he understood the immutable place of men and women in this world, had instilled in me an appreciation of the feminine. I grew from that point, always comfortable in a woman's company throughout my life, eager to cherish she who makes man complete.

Belinda saved the ring she had made for me in 1990, and we married in 1992. Now we are apart rarely, a week here, a few days now and again, but we never tire of each other's company. I hear no complaints about the demands my paralysis puts upon her. If we are angry with one another, we sit face to face, grasp hands, and speak openly of the hurt. I have told her of the pain, the desperation, the fear, the rejection inherent in being handled in anger, in being made to feel like an unwanted, overbearing obligation. She understands, I'm sure. She has said so. And she has acted so.

It is Belinda who slides me from bed to chair, chair to chair, and chair to bed.

It is Belinda who trims my toenails, gets up in the middle of the night when I need antacids, and watches my eyes for any pain I attempt to sublimate.

It is Belinda who quietly tends this thing that lives with us, this disability that sometimes fades away in the light of her love.

She says it will forever be so.

. . . .

By the time that we married, I already understood I'd been luckier than most people with disabilities. Nevertheless, I was greedy, and I wished—sometimes silently, sometimes aloud, but never with Belinda responding "If wishes were horses, beggars would ride"—that I could have been luckier still.

I could have been born to money. Money may not have kept me from getting polio, but money lessens the material constraints that are the frosting on the disability cake. Instead, my luck is of a different stripe. I'm a baby boomer born to people who fought their way out of the Great Depression and into the middle class. And there they taught their children early to make do, which is a decent mantra for coping with a disability.

But the lack of surplus money has also meant I've ridden through life without exotic, not-absolutely-necessary tools like electronic door systems, or whirlpool baths with electronic transfer lifts, or self-lowering vans equipped with zero-effort driving controls.

As the Duchess of Windsor once said, "You can never be too rich or too thin." The old girl was correct, about affluence and about the right physical shape if you intend to spend a lifetime using a wheelchair.

Thin, you're easy to lift. Rich, you can hire someone to lift you.

If the duchess had used a wheelchair long enough, she might have also learned there is one more essential quality to the life disabled: malleability.

Disability hammers, pounds, and bends. A person with a disability must be willing to change without breaking. I've motored around on my fanny long enough to know that the ability to adapt to that which cannot be changed is the key element in learning to live boob high to the world.

It also provides an interesting perspective.

The only beings I normally greet at eye level are children and large dogs. Since those are two of the nicer segments of the world's population, I don't complain. In a crowd or in a line, my view is of chests or backs. Accuse me of looking at a woman's bust line first, and I won't even try to make excuses.

Belinda is a delicate five feet six inches tall, and the words are her description, said with a teasing laugh—"boob high to the world." In my chair, I am fourteen inches shorter than her. That means she bends down and leans over to kiss me. Before we married, as we grew closer and the kisses moved from cheek to lip, there to linger and lengthen, I began to pull her toward me. I would rest my left hand below her ribcage and my right hand on the side of her face or the back of her neck.

Familiarity bred intimacy, and intimacy meant my left hand began to stray upward on a regular basis as we kissed.

"One of these days," Belinda said, "you're going to do that when another woman leans over to kiss you, and there'll be fireworks."

"Other women don't kiss me," I said.

"How about Mom?" she said. "Or Roxane," she continued, referring to her sister, "or Jon's wife?" With those three, and one or two touchy-feely female friends she added when I lifted my eyebrows in amusement, she named nearly every person with mammary glands whom I addressed by first name.

"I'll claim you taught me," I said, but inwardly decided it best that I clamp my hands together if I'm kissed by anyone except Belinda.

And so it is, here in the fifth decade of my paralysis, that I sit boob high to the world and content—a man no longer in the embrace of anger and self-pity and frustration, instead freed by love.

This woman, this Belinda, this Eve, broke open the shell of my loneliness and ignited passion, a passion that flowered into a spiritual connection, a connection that deepens each day we are together.

27

Belinda was the mother of two boys when we met—Matthew, age four, and Christopher, age six. When her husband, Tom, left, he had no desire to take his sons with him. He preferred to make threats about having her declared unsuitable because of her hearing impairment, a disability she had had since birth.

The threats, although no doubt empty, caused Belinda still more emotional turmoil. Intellectually, she understood Tom didn't want the responsibility of raising two children, but she felt herself in peril of losing her sons.

Belinda had coped adequately with her hearing impairment, at least after it was discovered. Her early inability to understand everything going on in her environment had caused her to act out, so much so that some experts advised her parents to consider institutionalizing her. Her mother refused. She decided to teach Belinda to speak correctly herself, a remarkable accomplishment for a woman who had married before completing high school. By the time the family had moved from Chicago to southwest Missouri, Belinda had reached the stage where, with the use of hearing aids and with remarkable personal energy, she was able to attend public school. She always ranked in the top ten percent of her classes.

She had married Tom Baldwin during the summer following her graduation from high school. She was nineteen, but, she has told me, "I was still a little girl."

Her attempt at building the marriage she wanted didn't last through the honeymoon, although it took more than six years before Tom left and a civil divorce was granted. Belinda was ambitious and Tom was obstructive. Tom was critical and Belinda was sensitive. Tom handled her roughly, using his physical superiority to attempt to dominate her, and Belinda said, "If you ever hit me, you better not go to sleep in this house."

Those half dozen years of turmoil, and her early struggles through her hearing impairment, had left Belinda with a near indomitable will to achieve and a hidden but sometimes overwhelming sense of inferiority. Once the shock over the collapse of her marriage began to fade, those two qualities came to the fore. She worried, she cried, but she persevered. She recognized that if she moved into the shelter of her family she might derail any chance for independence. And she realized that her boys expressed a need for a mother more than the companionship of an absent father, and so she set out to make the home the two youngsters needed and deserved.

After she rented a public housing apartment in the town where I lived, she began finding part-time work to fit around her duties as an adjunct instructor, her master's degree classes, and her thesis project. When that wasn't enough, she turned to student loans.

In spite of our deepening friendship, Belinda refused to take money from me. The only thing she allowed me to do was help with childcare when I wasn't at work myself. The grounds surrounding my apartment offered the boys trees to climb, space to ride bicycles, and room to run free.

The older boy, Christopher, was tall for his age and extremely lanky. He had his mother's brunette hair, dark eyes, and a voracious appetite. In spite of near-constant foraging through refrigerators and cupboards, he remained gangly and rawboned, a perfect child to dress up as Ichabod Crane on Halloween.

Matthew, the younger, was average-size for a four-year-old. He was a hyperactive redhead who heard only what he wanted to hear and cried when pressed to do anything against his will. Told to do something, or told to stop doing something, he was likely to scrunch up his green eyes in frustration he seemed unable to articulate and burst out crying. Both boys missed their father, or perhaps they missed the normalcy of a two-parent household.

Tom, mostly at the behest of his parents who enjoyed the boys' company, would stop by infrequently to pick them up for a weekend visit. Occasionally one or the other would refuse to accompany him, which I found odd, but not as odd as Tom's seeming indifference to the rejection. Most often it was Matthew, whose very arrival in this world had been a surprise to Tom.

Even though I tried to pull back from interacting with him, I came to think Tom was a man who knew before his marriage that he was making the wrong choice but didn't have the courage to face the truth. Belinda told me his first words on the church steps following the ceremony were "You're lucky I showed up."

Belinda was too strong, too stubborn, too ambitious to be fenced in by what she soon learned was Tom's parochial view of the world and a woman's place in it. He opposed her desire to attend college, but, once she had her degree, he had expected her to find a job and start bringing in a paycheck. And cook. And care for the boys. And keep house.

I admired Belinda's intellectual strength and emotional depth and the power of her will, but Tom apparently disliked or perhaps even feared those qualities in a woman.

Tom seemed to want nothing more than to work his three twelve-hour shifts in a food production plant and spend the remainder of his days playing. I learned he was the child of a second marriage, his father, I think, a retired military noncommissioned officer who had married a woman with two or three children. Tom liked to hunt, ride bicycles, and fancied himself a martial arts expert.

During this period, I sometimes referred to Tom as Doofus when talking about him with Belinda, regrettably sometimes even in the presence of his sons. I am ashamed of the harm that label inflicted on Chris and Matt, both of whom were doubtless in turmoil following the collapse of their home. I tried not to hate Tom for the wounds he had inflicted on Belinda, but I let my contempt for him show, and that was a sorrowful and lasting mistake, one I have since tried to amend in conversations with the boys.

Belinda had been introduced to Tom by her mother, one of Tom's co-workers. Had Belinda's mother thought her naïve and overly diffident daughter incapable of finding dating material? Perhaps, for Belinda had grown up sheltered and protected, and her hearing impairment isolated her from many of the boisterous activities of childhood and adolescence. Soon after we met, I began to realize Belinda was extraordinarily shy, especially in groups where the trickling noise of multiple conversations becomes a river's roar, an indecipherable din. Belinda also was skittish because of previous romantic experiences, with one or two of her early encounters with boys resulting in being pushed too far, too fast.

"I don't know why I married Tom," Belinda once told me. "I guess because I wanted to get out of the house. No one believed in me—believed I could accomplish becoming a scientist. The trouble was Tom lied about believing in me."

I loved my mother unconditionally. I loved my father, respected the power of his will and his stoicism, his loyalty and his protective nature, fearing only his anger and disapproval. I love my brother, admire his accomplishments, and honor the blood-tie between us. I love Belinda, my wife, with appreciation for her femininity, with admiration for her intellect and spiritual depth, and with the secret dark lust of the primal male pinning the eternal female to him.

But how do you love a child not your own?

I can remember a Sunday, the first one after Labor Day. Early September can be a mellow time in southern Missouri, and the four of us were attending a group picnic. Shortly before the buffet was opened, I glanced down a little incline leading from the picnic shelter toward a set of playground equipment. Matthew, eight years old, had himself wrapped around the leg of a boy almost twice his size and age, while Christopher was alternately swinging wildly and dodging blows directed at him by the same teenager. I set off down the slope in my power chair, intent on ramming my way into the middle of the skirmish.

"Hey, kid!" I yelled. "Find someone your own size to pick on!" The struggle stopped.

"And you two," I said, pointing at Chris and Matt, "get your butts back up to the pavilion and try to stay out of trouble for a few minutes."

Belinda's father had told her she shouldn't marry me because a man in a wheelchair couldn't be a good father for her boys. He was right, but not in the way he thought, not because I couldn't play catch with them or help them build a tree house. It had nothing to do with the wheelchair, not in a direct sense. Granted, I am what the wheelchair has made me, this man too rigidly protective of self, too closed off sometimes to understand how to open his heart. But with all that, with all the warped qualities of my wheelchair personality, I think my failures as a substitute father had more to do with my Pavlovian mimicking of my father's parenting techniques. I preferred rules to listening, and I felt disappointed when Chris and Matt failed to live out my own thwarted ambitions.

It was the me who lives inside this hulk who could not grow into what a father should be, who now like every other man responsible for a child's welfare looks back and only wants to do it again better. The wheelchair was irrelevant or at least could have been made so.

In fact, at first the wheelchair was an attraction. Matt was small enough that he would demand to ride in my lap when we shopped at a mall, went to a theme park, or visited other attractions. I allowed Chris to alternate early on, but he soon outgrew both my lap and the desire to ride.

Sometimes when Belinda would work the night shift, the boys would sleep on the sofa bed in my apartment. Although I'm certain Belinda related the circumstances of my paralysis to them in a manner they could comprehend, I found their response interesting as they began to see with their own eyes that I needed help with some of the simpler functions of living. Early on, Chris would often rush to grab my legs as I was being lifted into bed by one of the personal care attendants I had hired. I was surprised at this reaction—Instinct? Currying favor? Simply the desire to be involved?

My brother, Jon, only eight when I was paralyzed, had been somewhat isolated from the demands for care I made on the people around me. Although I never asked, I believe it was a conscious decision on my parents' part. I was their child. They would take care of me. I would not be a burden to my brother.

What does it teach a child to be pulled into the orbit of a person with a disability? Looking now at Jon, who silently assumed the right to help me in response to the obligations of blood and heart, and looking at the young men Chris and Matt have grown into, I believe it teaches empathy. Chris and Matt had a head start even before they were deposited in my life. They learned early that their mother had trouble with certain sounds, especially when emitted by a television or radio. They began to interpret for her, no doubt even before they comprehended the reasons for her questions. As their little family moved into my world, they seemed to understand that I could not reach or lift certain things. It became second nature for them to assist me, not because I asked, but because it had to be done.

As my relationship with Belinda deepened, the boys began to spend most of their time with me, sometimes even overnight, with Belinda coming in late from work or school to crash on the sofa. Chris, Matt, and I soon evolved into cooks and housekeepers, taking care of ourselves and even of Belinda as she devoted her energy to working and studying. Though I continued working part-time at an insurance agency, I could help prepare the boys for school and be available when they returned home. We soon discovered that one advantage of small-town life is that it made a trip to the nearby grocery store easy: a guy in a power chair trailed by two boys on bicycles; the boys reach for objects on high shelves, pack the sacks, and help carry them home.

We were a family even before Belinda and I married on February 29, 1992. Chris was eight. Matt was six. We bought a dusty-rose-colored brick house on a corner opposite a church parsonage in Aurora, acquired a mortgage, a dog, and a lawnmower, and then began to learn that a good marriage was far easier to accomplish than raising two boys to adulthood without problems.

It didn't take long for us to begin recognizing that Chris was waltzing through school on charm, finding high marks easy to earn by courting his teachers. He never found a real focus in elementary or high school—not science, not mathematics, not language. When he was a junior, he took a part-time job in a fast-food franchise, eventually working up to a shift manager's position. It mirrored his interest in cooking at home. More to the point, it mirrored his lifelong interest in food.

Neither Belinda nor I had big appetites, focusing our kitchen activities mostly on attempting to see that the boys had assorted meats and vegetables and a limited number of sweets. I liked finger food. She liked chicken and chocolate kisses. I drank tea. She drank diet soda. But as the boys grew, we learned the economy of visiting the all-you-can-eat buffet restaurants simply to satisfy their appetites, Chris's in particular.

Upon graduation from high school, Chris used the free credits earned by the state A-Plus Program—payment for college tuition in return for maintaining a specific grade average and participating in extracurricular activities—to enroll for a culinary arts degree at a local community college. The effort seemed a natural choice.

But, close to obtaining his degree in culinary arts, Chris found the restaurant business wasn't the sort of work he wanted to do for a lifetime, and he enrolled in a university in pursuit of a degree in sports medicine or sports nutrition. Chris married in 2006, and he now journeys toward that place in life where two men—Tom and me—failed him in ways we did not choose. If he's lucky, his mistakes will be his own, and he will be a better man, a better father, for it.

Conversely, Matt grew to be the problem child. There's blame enough—and more than sufficient guilt—for Tom, for Belinda, and for me, although none of us understands completely what guidance we might have provided to save Matthew from himself. Looking back, I know the nature of free will and the open-ended idea of personal responsibility dominates most lives, but I will never comprehend what makes a first-grade teacher, a woman esteemed in church and community, tell the parents of a child, "If you don't get control of him, he's going to be a criminal."

What did the woman see that we did not? What did we miss?

True, Matt was hard to handle, crying in frustration when I sat with him for hours to help him learn to read. And reading wasn't the only reason he seemed to care nothing for school. He simply scraped by, never being held back in spite of learning little, even with summer school sessions and constant help at home. He thought of school as nothing more than a play date.

Each year his behavior and his willingness to learn deteriorated further. He wanted to go to school, but he had no conception it was a place to learn, to prepare for a self-sufficient life. We asked for tests, and he was diagnosed with a possible attention deficit disorder. A physician tried a course of Ritalin. There were no changes.

We were confused because Matt was relatively well behaved at home, boyishly lazy about chores, intent on video games when allowed, able to memorize extraordinary amounts of media trivia but unable to remember—or care about—chores and responsibilities. That cavalier attitude applied to school obligations and homework, no matter who nagged or how much. When he was sent to the principal, he would smile, agree, and promise to do better. Belinda and I were called in to discuss his situation first with teachers and administrators and then with counselors. Not one believed our reports of his acceptable behavior at home. In fact, although we understood he was childish and required attentive supervision, we thought Matt's behavior at home outshone what we observed among the children of acquaintances.

"Would you like a .22 rifle, Matt?" we asked when he brought home a series of failing grades on his first high school report card. "We know Tom promised Chris one, and we think you could handle one too."

"Sure," he replied. For reasons lurking below the surface, in spite of the fact that Belinda and I always provided identical gifts, Matt always felt as if he lived in Chris's shadow.

"Bring home passing grades next quarter, and we'll buy you one."

His enthusiasm lasted a week or perhaps two. We saw a handful of sloppily written papers with a teacher's "Much better!" scribbled across them in red ink, but then there came another call from the school with another problem to report.

Nothing worked, not even psychological counseling or a sojourn in a residential unit for troubled adolescents, after Matt had disappeared from home for three days. We called the police and reported him missing. He then showed up on his own, but he had self-inflicted cuts on his arms. The counselor recommended the residential center, and we enrolled him immediately. When he was released after six months, Matt decided we were the problem. "I'm going to live with my real dad," he said. He was sixteen.

His decision came in response to justifiable discipline after a major crisis—once again, Matt had disappeared for two days; this time he was suffering badly from the aftereffects of binge drinking.

"It was Friday the 13th—that's freak night—I went out with some friends to celebrate," he told us. He seemed confused that we did not understand that young people had the right to party, as he put it, even if it happened to get out of hand—such as an older youth providing alcohol to an immature sixteen-year-old.

Matt left, and then a few months later left his father's house in a dispute with his stepmother, and then finally dropped out of school altogether. After a scrape with the legal system, he returned to our house full of remorse, and his brother found him a job as a cook in the fast-food restaurant where he was assistant manager. We helped him enroll in general education degree courses. He left again and came home in desperation once more. And then left again. And returned once more, this time after moving in with a group of supposed friends who urged him to co-sign a lease, demand he pay them cash for a share of living expenses, and finally left him to account for unpaid bills.

Matt, now in his early twenties, lives down the hall from the bedroom Belinda and I share, working steadily at a local automobile dealer, moving among a group of acquaintances who, like him, struggle with the complexities of the modern world.

Saved from rejection because somewhere deep in his heart is an element of gentleness and goodness, Matt floats through life, working hard to connect his ambitions to the level of energy necessary to achieve them. He's received Missouri's General Equivalency Diploma and enrolled for a few classes in a technical college. Belinda helped him organize his finances so that he could buy a small parcel of wooded acreage without making a down payment. On weekends, he hops in his rusted old pickup and drives out to the acreage, working to clear the land with a chain saw. He dreams of building a house that looks like a castle.

I keep silent.

. . . .

"People are weird," Matt told me this past year. He had been working part-time in an all-night restaurant to supplement his income. "There's this new girl, a waitress, and a couple of our regulars came in. The woman uses a walker. Her husband is in a wheelchair. The new girl wouldn't wait on them."

"I don't know what to say. They make me nervous," the new waitress had told Matt.

"What's to say?" he had replied. "Treat them like any other customer. They don't want anything from you except to write down their order and bring their food."

For all the failures I feel as a parent—for my lack of empathy and respect for the boys' father, for being overly strict at times and too lenient at others, for not finding some way to inspire either of them to latch onto a passion to pursue—I think both Chris and Matt have learned at least to see disability as simply one color in the spectrum of the human condition.

When they came into my life, each with a child's natural inquisitiveness, I always answered the questions sparked by that curiosity, talking openly about my disability and replying truthfully. They understood early on the reason I use a wheelchair and the reason I would need to do so the remainder of my life. And they understood that using a wheelchair is not the most perfect way to travel through the world. But I have never heard either of them voice fears about their own well-being or health. I was a man in a wheelchair, and they were free to run and play. Over time, they learned to offer help only when circumstances warranted, understanding that my wheelchair afforded independence and a degree of liberation from paralysis, and understanding that too much help, unrequested help, lessens independence. My wheelchair, my disability, was normal in their world, a world where I worked, wrote, interacted with friends, and loved their mother.

Chris, Matt, and I now treat one another with respect, we three males with the closest relationship to the woman who brought us together, the woman whom we all cherish. I have learned a little more each day that Chris and Matt are not me; that my ambitions, likes, and dislikes have no place in the lives they are free to choose for themselves.

They call me Dad, and I try to offer advice that helps but does not interfere. That's all that we can ask of each other.

We make our choices, and the world spins out of our control anyway. I wanted Belinda. Dear God, I could not keep myself from marrying her. Blinded by loneliness and aching with desire, I used her need to fill my need, pulling her into my orbit with the power of the passion I felt for her. I am only sorry I did not find the wisdom earlier to treasure enough the gifts she brought with her—two vital young boys.

28

Shortly after we first met, before we engaged in that dance where friends become lovers and lovers become husband and wife, Belinda told me, "I'm a cradle Catholic." I knew what that meant in spite of having attended church rarely during my adult life.

While Belinda was, in fact, baptized into the church as an infant, she hadn't attended Mass regularly until she earned her driver's license and began to go to church by herself. That curiosity marked her first step in what has become a lifelong exploration to find meaning and purpose in life.

I understood from the first that the Roman Catholic Church was important to her, so significant that it even colored the way she voiced her perception of her failing marriage. "One thing I think helps is that we're both Catholic," she had told me a few days after we met. I had asked an innocuous question about her family life. There was no hint in her reply that she and Tom had been sleeping in separate bedrooms for several years. Neither was there an admission that Tom had only joined the church during their courtship to appease her.

One day, perhaps a year after we found each other, Belinda asked me if I would like to go to Mass with her. I remember now being nervous, mostly because I would be meeting people I had known for years through business or community activities in an unfamiliar setting—almost an exclusive club, in fact. Only a small percentage of people in southern Missouri are Roman Catholic, and, in the little town where I lived—and where Belinda had moved after her civil divorce—fewer than two hundred families were members of the Catholic church.

In the isolated Ozark hills settled by Anglo-Saxons and Celt descendants migrating from Appalachia, Roman Catholics had once been perceived as idol-worshipers. The French and Spanish had brought Catholicism to the parts of Missouri along the Mississippi River, but the Church never penetrated the lost nation in the state's southwest corner. Aurora, in fact, had been the home of a racist, anti-Catholic newspaper, *The Menace*, in the early twentieth century. Thus, the local Catholic church, Holy Trinity, was a tight-knit community made up of descendants of German and Polish immigrants who came to the hills half a century or more after the original settlers.

I had never liked church—practical, organized religious worship in the midst of a group led by a charismatic speaker. When I agreed to attend a Saturday evening Mass with Belinda, I expected a cool reception at best or outright rejection at worst. Instead, I found myself surprised at the attitude of the local priest and the people making up the congregation of Holy Trinity. My welcome was quiet and sincere. I found my presence accepted without question, and there was no pressure to make a decision to convert or to join, a process I was soon to learn was far more complicated than the country practice of answering an altar call.

My journey toward the Catholic faith began poorly, even boorishly on my part. There were probably thirty parishioners present when we made our entrance. Heads began to turn my way immediately as the sound of my power chair echoed from the vaulted ceiling. I greeted everyone I knew as we moved toward an empty pew.

"Hey, Charlie."

A nod in return.

"Joe, good to see you."

Another nod.

Belinda and I found an empty pew, and, as she knelt to say her prayers, she leaned toward my chair and said, "We're supposed to be quiet and reverent when we enter church, sweetie."

In spite of my initial ill manners, people made a point of greeting me after the service. The warm reception wasn't a fluke. As our months together passed, Belinda sometimes attended Mass alone or with the boys, but soon we began attending as a family. Each time we went to worship together—this lonely divorced woman in a church that does not recognize divorce, accompanied by her solitary, too often cynical companion, friend, and lover—we found acceptance. It seemed as if there would always be room at Holy Trinity for one more seeker, one more sinner.

No one at Holy Trinity asked me if I had been saved—that is, accepted Jesus Christ as Lord and Savior, the declaration of faith common to many Protestant denominations—but I had, once long ago, in a dark, solitary hospital room, in an iron lung, in peril of living only one more day, or two, at the most.

It was the year of my transformation, my first days, in fact, in the polio ward in 1959. The stranger who entered my room that fall night had been dressed all in white. I had been in the iron lung for a number of days I can no longer remember, and the stranger in white said he could save me. I was raging with fever, and I had lost track of time and of nearly everything that was happening around me, to me. I only knew I was in a hospital, and I was seriously ill.

"Do you know Jesus is your only hope?" the man asked. "Your Lord and Savior?" When the question came, I believed I was already being saved. Weren't the doctors doing their best? I was still alive, right?

"What do you mean?" I asked. It was nighttime, black outside and lights off inside, and the man had simply walked into my room, carrying no tray, no device, bearing instead the invisible determination to win a soul for Jesus. White man, in white slacks, white short-sleeved shirt. I assumed he was an orderly or a hospital technician of some sort. I had been awake, eyes focused on the hallway waiting for something to appear there or in my dreams. The man may have introduced himself, but his abrupt question chased his name out of my mind.

It didn't scare me, the question. I had been knocked down by polio and kicked around by pneumonia, but I still wore the armor of youthful ignorance. I knew I was in the middle of a mess, but I wasn't afraid I would die. People around me may have thought so, but not me. No, not me.

"Jesus died for your sins. He has bought the whole world a place in heaven if we'll just accept Him as Lord and Savior. You'd like that, wouldn't you?"

"I guess . . ." I said, thinking mostly about the man's use of the word *bought*.

The stranger stood at the head of the iron lung, the light from the hallway reflecting from his white uniform. His face remained shadowed. He talked about his church, asked briefly about my family, and then once again declared the only hope for me lay in my desire to give my soul to Jesus. And then he left.

My visitor's pastor, a Baptist minister from one of the larger churches in Springfield, came the next morning, saying he'd been told about my situation. That meant more talk. He was a man about my father's age, nattily dressed in a blue pin-striped suit. His dark wavy hair was being chased off the top of his head. He carried a well-worn Bible, and he relished the victory of another lost soul being snatched from the snares of Beelzebub.

It took only a minute for the minister to fixate on the importance of being saved. I felt confused, but eager to please, and I knew the idea was certainly important to the visitor in white and to the preacher who came at his bidding, people who apparently had gone out of their way for my benefit. We prayed, the wavy-haired reverend and me. Then there were thanks and congratulations.

If there was a big change in my life, I took it lying down.

I was surprised that afternoon at my father's reaction when I told him about my night visitor and the pastor who followed in his wake.

"What do you mean?" my father asked when I said the orderly was worried about me being saved. "That's not his business. And you don't need to worry about it now. You need to concentrate on getting well. That's all. They need to leave you alone."

"But they care about my soul." I was puzzled. I thought it interesting that two strangers were worried, that I was that important to people I didn't know at all.

I couldn't understand my father's anger, which seemed equally divided between the idiocy of a teenage boy being so corrupt that his soul was in peril and the idea of two strangers believing they had the right to approach a critically ill adolescent with the news that he was in danger of hell. I had always known that my father thought there was an inviolable wall around his private life, even if the world didn't. And I knew he wasn't much on organized religion. I was certain he believed God ruled the universe, but I think he lost any appreciation for love and mercy, for God's better angels walking among mankind, in the battle for the island of Okinawa.

"Don't you think I do?" His green eyes always opened wide and turned to steel when I defied his judgment. "And your mother? We care about you—more than these people, that's for sure—and what we want is for people to leave you alone so that you can get well."

Long afterward, I began to appreciate the deeper nuances of what my father did not articulate then. It was after I began to see the line between concern for the soul of your fellow man and the manipulation of someone weak, ravaged, and defenseless.

That happened only after I began to think more clearly about life, about the abstract and tenuous hold that each of us has on our existence, whether we are whole or maimed. It was then that religion—not church, but rather the mystical and intellectual conception of the Divine—became for me a melding of mind and spirit. It was a time when I began to read agnostics and atheists like Carl Sagan and Stephen Hawking and to think about life and self-awareness flowering in this isolated corner of the Infinite.

I thought back to the stranger in white, and I understood he had not been wrong, at least as he conceived God's place in his world, but rather that he had misread why we had been drawn together, that he had such a nebulous grip on the idea of reflecting God's will that what transpired became less than holy. Confused, perhaps even frightened, I was left to stare at the ceiling paralyzed and puzzled while the stranger in white walked away with another star for the heavenly crown he felt awaited him.

It was years before I remembered the lesson I learned while lying afraid, listening to the man in white and his shepherd a few hours later. It is a simple one, really, about silent prayers for grace and for the will to live on one more minute, hour, day, content with the holy mystery held out by God for His creation to contemplate. I learned it only at the end of a long period during which I lived almost alone in the world, surrounded by acquaintances rather than friends, and learned it again when I married and converted to Catholicism. God's own miracle, those blessed unions.

When I began attending Mass with Belinda, I found that, as much as fundamentalism adheres to the certainty of eternal damnation, Catholicism meditates on the everlasting prospect of reconciliation and redemption—the rightness of God's creation. Astrophysicists may preach that we live in a four-dimensional world drifting in five-dimensional space, and evangelists may cry out we reek with the ugliness of original sin, but it is left to us, alone in the night, to face our puzzling complexity: eternally adrift in creation, journeying from a place of preexistence toward a nonplace outside of space, time, matter, energy.

We within the One, Holy, Catholic, and Apostolic Church meditate upon enigma.

As our immersion into the community of Holy Trinity continued, Belinda filed for an annulment of her marriage to Tom. "I want to get married in the church again," she told me.

That marked the point I began to consider joining the Catholic Church—not because of the infallibility of the pope, the man who sits on Peter's rock, and not because a confession to a priest might absolve me from every failure. Rather, it began as Belinda and I talked about the foundation the church provided for her life as a woman, as a child of God.

I also joined because of the dreams of long ago, the dreams of a hundred or more nights, when the shadows and ghosts of what I had been lingered in the night, in a place where I first explored the dark world of disability that had descended upon me, in the fantasies where I lived whole and imagined I would marry a woman of the Catholic faith.

As St. Joan mused, how else would God speak to us but in dreams?

Over the months and years, Belinda and I received generous help in our quest to become one within the church. She yearned for annulment, a recognition by those who shared her beliefs that she had entered into a one-sided commitment—a promise unfulfilled, a covenant made with a deceiver—when she offered her vows at the ceremony that supposedly bound her to Thomas Baldwin. Belinda received assistance with the long, complicated bureaucratic process from a lay church worker who had known her for several years, including the period when Belinda sought out counseling and support as her marriage crumbled around her.

The help I received came in the form of acceptance and instruction, first from Father Peter, a Polish priest—a native of Silesia, actually, whose older brother had been drafted into the Wehrmacht as a medic and killed by the Allies—who had left his country to help fill a clerical void in the United States. A small man, gray-haired, quick-moving, tight-lipped, and not always sure of his command of English, Father Peter was popular with his congregation. A cynic might have guessed the generous opinion was sparked by his ten-minute homilies, sermons remarkably shorter than those from priests who had grown up speaking English. But even a casual observer soon understood that behind the language barrier and beneath the collar lived a true servant, a gentle man who loved the church. No one spoke ill of Father Peter.

At our first meeting, after he greeted Belinda, he reached down, grabbed my hand, and said "And your name? What it is?"

Father Peter, in fact, carried a car insurance account at the agency where I worked, but I don't think he recognized me in the unfamiliar setting of the church's foyer. I waited quietly after I gave him my name, anticipating the familiar questions a Protestant pastor might ask.

"Do you know the Lord Jesus—are you saved? Where's your church home?"

Father Peter simply released my hand, touched my shoulder, and said "God bless." Then he moved on to another person waiting to greet him.

After I began to attend Mass regularly, he invariably made it a point to greet me, acting as if it was the most natural thing in the world for me to want to attend Mass with Belinda. Then, a year after our marriage, when I told him I would like to be baptized into the church, he merely nodded and said, "I make arrangements."

I have attended Mass in cathedrals and in churches big and small, but I have never been as embraced by the sense of brotherhood, of fellowship, as I was at Holy Trinity. There I sat in the warmth of God's house and listened as His words described the nature of love—for family, for one another, for the world—the resolution of conflict without violence, feeding the hungry and sheltering the poor, and celebrating life as it ignites in the womb and forever locking the doors of the death chamber.

"Would you like me to join the Church?" I had asked Belinda. We were in our second year of marriage, attending together as a family. Her annulment request had been granted, and Father Peter had pronounced us husband and wife in a quiet ceremony attended by family.

"Don't join for me," she replied. "I made that mistake once. Join only if it is important to you."

And so I did. First, baptism, with Belinda as my sponsor and my brother and his family, Methodists all, watching from the front pew quietly, as if they did not know what to make of the man who sought the holy waters, or of the one who might emerge. And then Confirmation, the lone adult, seated and silent, among jittery, bubbling teenagers kneeling and rising to take the last step toward unity with the saints of the ages.

The bishop stepped down and asked my confirmation name. "John," I said. The bishop didn't need to know which one, but I had chosen it in honor of my brother, in apology and in love, and in pursuit of a mystical connection with John the Baptist, that prophet so sure, so fervent, so filled with the power of all that is holy that Salome recoiled in horror when presented with his head.

And so I began a life of communion with the church, began searching through the transcendental teachings of a simple Jewish carpenter, among a congregation He gave over to Peter, the Rock. I feel at home in the Roman Catholic Church because I believe it is old enough and secure enough—it might even be said, rich enough—to accept the world as it is and yet act every day to make it better. And I like that. I can approach a priest, a man with no investment in anything other than his vows, without being judged. I can enter any church, sit quietly, and contemplate the unfathomable idea that Infinite Truth descends to the altar when the priest raises the Host toward heaven.

Father Peter, and his quiet acceptance of this thing I am, was assigned to another congregation shortly after my conversion. Father Allan Saunders was his replacement, another priest with a gentle, accepting understanding that we, priest and parishioner alike, are wayward pilgrims searching for the road home.

Father Allan became friend and mentor to both Belinda and me. We often had him to dinner or invited him to go to the movies with us.

"I get so damn angry," I have told Father Allan. "And, yeah, I know. You're going to say anger is a form of self-pity."

There's a trace of Protestantism still at the edge of my soul, and I sometimes cannot separate the Sacrament of Reconciliation from personal counseling, but Father Allan seems to hear the questions I don't ask as I stumble toward an elusive peace with the person I have become.

Father Allan usually replies, "Everyone gets angry."

"I'd rather be at peace, not be forced to chew on frustration every day."

"Who wouldn't?"

"But I watch you at the altar. You raise the Host, and the Cup, and I envy your belief. I expect your hands to glow as the accident of bread becomes . . ."

"Sometimes you must act like you believe before you can believe," he says.

I think about all the healers and heathens I have drawn into my orbit. And when I close my eyes and rest my head in my hands, remembering a lifetime of holy mysteries, I know I will always be welcome in the Catholic Church, a community of believers and pretenders, failures and posers, all watched over by a Christ who'll rise once more and forever and walk to His destiny.

. . . .

I am a Catholic who cannot kneel. Instead, after we have found a pew, it is my habit to pick up the missal, the little book outlining the order of worship, while Belinda drops to her knees and says her prayers. One Sunday not long after I had joined the Church, the day's order of worship was introduced with a meditation that concluded with the sentence, "God grant that we might dwell in the holy mystery of our lives, not needing to know the future so much as willing to live each day fully and gracefully, through Christ who sets us free."

"Read this," I said to Belinda when she arose and sat in the pew.

"Beautiful, isn't it?" she replied after digesting the sentence.

I pulled out my wallet, found a scrap of paper, and began to write out the sentence. I memorized it. I wrote the words into a computer screen saver that floats, illuminated, before me when I pause in my writing.

Such is my Catholicism—a belief narrowed down from the pope in Rome and all the glorious cathedrals raised in the name of the Carpenter, down to the prayer I have crafted from those words, words shaped into a plea for individual grace and the acceptance of holy mysteries.

I find joy and peace and truth in those words, and cling to them with much more faith than the mantra I embraced even before I became paralyzed, the ancient stoic paradigm *This too shall pass*. Each transcendental truth has worked its magic, although differently, as I have rolled through life, experiencing the accidental riding lessons necessary for me to make this long journey on wheels.

I spent years, decades, believing *This too shall pass* without ever asking *Into what?* More of the same, it seemed, at least as I rolled through the years of my twenties and thirties.

Stoicism was a natural mindset for me. I had been taught from the words of my father that endurance outweighs complaint—that things were as they were because they had been ordained by time or custom.

Is there logic behind the catastrophic damage to my physical body, behind the collision of my healthy body with a random virus? In the absence of reason, how else could I embrace paralysis other than immersion in stoicism?

Do I now embrace the faith that the universe unfolds as the Eternal Creator directs simply because there is no other rationale?

I know that only after I accepted the idea that grace flows down on every living creature did I then begin to think of myself as something other than a person with a disability, to learn to care less that I live my days in a wheelchair, to understand that within the holy mystery of my life the wheelchair has never defined me.

29

A few years after Belinda and I married, after I had accepted the faith that had cradled her, I began to write articles and essays regarding issues of disability in the community and in the church. I sent opinion pieces to regional newspapers. I signed on as disability issues editor for a section of a prominent Web site. I had always written, using the act of striking a keyboard as a mechanism to expand the way I thought about the world and my place in it. The passion had begun with the old Underwood my father bought me as a tool to restore my dexterity after I returned home from the rehabilitation center in 1960. It continued with dozens of notebooks filled with random thoughts, lists of books I had read, and incidents at the office worth remembering.

I had kept all those words private. Nevertheless, especially after I began to write about life as a person with a disability, I found myself speaking out even if what I said or published sometimes hurt feelings.

"I admire the bravery of Toni here, and Gary," said Holy Trinity's new pastor, Father Harold. "It takes courage to spend each day confined to a wheelchair."

I cringed. Belinda squeezed my hand. Father Allan, our friend and priest, had been sent to a parish in Missouri's bootheel.

"We look at the tiny crosses we who can walk are asked to bear," he continued, "and compare them to the cross each of our two friends here carries. Toni and Gary become inspirations to us."

Mass ended, and the congregation filed into the community hall for the traditional post-service coffee and doughnuts. "Do you mind if we stay until most people leave?" I asked Belinda. "I want to talk to Father Harold about his homily."

"I don't care," she replied. "Don't hurt his feelings, though. He meant well."

But I did. I pushed too hard, became too personal. I talked at him. I lectured, I suppose, trying to pound into him the difference between disability and illness, trying to make him understand that a person in a wheelchair should not be burdened with the idea that he must inspire others with his courage. I told him that riding in a wheelchair does not embellish a person's character. I tried to explain that there is a subtle denigration of humanity implicit when one person pities another.

"I don't want to be—I *can't* be—an example of bravery, Father Harold," I said. "It's not fair to assign me that responsibility. All I want—all anyone with a disability should want—is a chance, which in most cases means access and mechanisms that assure equal opportunity. A bonus would be for people to keep their prejudices to themselves."

I hurt Father Harold's feelings, and he never became my friend, but I will not refuse to speak out when I see prejudice sneer at the crips of this world, or when a person with a disability doesn't get a fair chance, or when the mangled, marred, and mutilated are met with pity rather than respect for their accomplishments. I hurt Father Harold's feelings because I felt his observation was based on pity.

As a crip who has learned to observe himself and his environment, I am amused by the black comedy staged when I motor about in public and listen to the internal dialogue ricocheting. I can almost see the thought processes of the people I meet, the words hanging over them like so many cartoon balloons.

"If I got stuck in a wheelchair, I'd shoot myself."

When I see that look, that flush of dark fearful recognition that life maims and kills, I almost want to pause and say, "Damned if I don't know what you mean."

30

The man who is Gimp will admit to finding disability boring.

That's a precipice I approach warily, for boredom leads to frustration, frustration to anger, and anger has a bastard son called self-pity, a malcontent who spawns little demons of hatred.

Hate. For self. For circumstance. Hate, corrosive hate. And hate kills. Trust me. I have looked behind that door.

Why boredom? For reasons simultaneously petty and pervasive. I am bored with living in Criptown because it takes me five minutes to slip on my winter coat, because I need to fetch a broomstick and knock an item off a top shelf if someone has left it in the wrong place, and because people don't really have anything new to say as I ride through my fifth decade in a wheelchair.

"I'm going to need one of those run-abouts soon," I hear from someone passing me in a store. "I have rheumatoid arthritis, and the pain is nearly unbearable during winter."

And so . . .

What? I have nothing to offer in return but a bland smile and an innocuous remark . . . unless you want me to dive into the dark depths of my soul where the rage shark swims. I would prefer not to take that plunge, and so instead I say, "Maybe that arthritis will improve once spring gets here."

And, yes, I know you have a relative who uses a chair just like mine, I reply to another person.

Yes, it's true we can always find someone worse off, I nod in response to the ancient bromide.

But there's one abrupt question I sometimes cannot dismiss with a casual shrug and a simple platitude.

"Hey, why are you in that wheelchair?"

Only small children can ask that question of me and get a fair answer, one I always attempt to fit to their ability to comprehend. Their mothers are invariably embarrassed, but I don't mind. I smile and open the child's eyes to the magic in my world.

And I usually don't mind that same sort of directness from the elderly either, although sometimes they probe deeper, and I must phrase the shots-gave-me-polio story in a way that won't result in me talking about it all day.

I am bored until I meet someone who cannot recognize personhood before disability. Then I refuse to allow my disability—Gimp, my Self—to become invisible. It's here. It's a normal part of life. I deal with it. You can deal with it too.

Then I tend to act out rather than speak up, so says my wife, who took psychology in college. I didn't go to college, but I have been known to give out psychology lessons on the streets.

Gimp once used my wheelchair to move a man ten or twenty feet, pushing him an inch at a time, because he insisted on standing in front of me at a public event. I could see nothing. He had entered the building long after I had selected a place to sit, parking beside a grandstand aisle to gain a clear view of my niece's high school graduation ceremony. As the crowd grew, this fellow gradually shuffled into my line of sight until he totally obscured my view.

The obvious answer? "Pardon me. Could you move slightly, please? I can't see."

Not me. Not the Gimp-invisible, not the imperceptible crip, not the guy who was there first and was sitting a mere ten inches away from his creased-khaki-clad ass.

I am Gimp. See me cope.

I eased my wheelchair forward until there was the slightest whisper of a touch of the metal footplates against his ankles, right where shoe top meets Achilles tendon. He moved forward an inch or so. I paused and then crept up again, smoothly, silently. Another tender kiss of metal upon the Achilles, that mythic place of vulnerability. Again, a step forward by the man who would not see. And then Gimp, once more, forward into the breech. Another gentle nudge.

I must have bumped his ankles ten or fifteen times. He never turned to see what nibbled at his feet. Gimp said nothing. The man said nothing. His wife trailing at his side said nothing. Me bumping ankles, moving from irritation over being invisible to curiosity over what I must do to be seen.

We waltzed silently, three inches here, four inches there, across the concrete floor to the music of cheers and the intermittent blasts of air horns, not for our parade but rather for the happy young people marching across the stage. Finally, the school board president called my niece's name, and I moved to where I could catch a glimpse of her as she stepped up to receive her diploma.

"A classic passive-aggressive action driven by repressed anger."

Thank you, doctor. I know.

But, dear God, it was fun, this malevolent experiment, this bizarre hunt for the elusive recognition of my personhood in the great forest of normalcy.

I marked it as an exploration of uncharted territory of criptology, the study of wheeled-beings interacting with an overwhelmingly biped environment.

. . . .

I am Gimp, invalid in your sight and wheelchair-bound in your fears—yes, yes, even if that which ties me to my chair is intangible. But among people of a certain age, people hard-worn and slow-moving, people who attend little churches and have big hearts, I hear promises of freedom.

"Your legs'll work in heaven, boy. Jesus will heal you, heal us all, and we'll walk the golden streets together up there."

Jesus loves them and me. The Bible tells me so. You need not believe. I only believe I understand, at least intellectually. And I believe in the mystic Truth of creation and in all the saints who proclaimed the Word.

And I believe in Gimp, the man who strives never to be cruel or sarcastic when someone carrying the weight of seven decades of sorrow and disappointment offers an empathy sandwich to nourish my spirit.

I am Gimp, and I appreciate irony, and I often find myself wheeling indifferently along the deep but narrow precipice between accepting what cannot be tolerated and ignoring what cannot be acknowledged. I am Gimp, willing now to ride out this life without complaint.

The cliché tells us life is unfair. I say it is also confusing. Should I care whether you approach me out of insincere pity, treacly sympathy, or true empathy?

"I pity you for being in that wheelchair."

What can I say in response?

"I pity you for not being able to understand that this wheelchair sets me free."

But it's all so damned confusing, that murky line between compassion and pity, sympathy and condescension. I only know one thing as dead certain as the polio-killed nerves in my spine. Pity is objectification. Count on that. And I know when I'm being pitied.

Why? Because I cringe at the idea of being robbed of my conception of the person I have constructed in this decades-long building project. Sincere sympathy may be a little better, but I don't want it. Whatever warmth it provides you, it is of no value to me. Empathy, silent empathy, that unvoiced assumption of our commonality, I suppose is best of all. Empathy does not ask me to decide if I am worthy. Empathy simply recognizes we all ride this world together, and, like mine, all of your conceptions about life, death, and disability are mere smudge marks on a dull gray sliding scale. I cannot find a place to mark off what I know, where knowledge ends and faith begins. I suppose you cannot either.

I am Gimp, a burnt-out case, and I must admit I am not interested in how you perceive me, how my broken carcass inspires your emotions.

I am Gimp, an embodiment of your fears and mine, an absurd hodgepodge of broken parts, reconstructed and miswired, sparking still, careening around in your comfort zone, knocking down your preconceptions and rolling over your hidden terrors.

I am Gimp, a creature more like you than you want me to be. For me, the line between ability and disability was drawn in my seventeenth year, and it glared solid, distinct, and perfectly fixed, much like the chalky circumscription wherein the crime-scene corpse once rested.

Outside the line was the new me, more helpless than a baby who arrives on this earth screaming in protest against his ejection from all that is familiar. Like the baby, I was ignorant of all that awaited. Hidden in the shadows sat Gimp, waiting patiently, a clone, disillusioned and deceived, eager to mock the weakling, the crippled creature newly born.

The promises made by old me, that boy's ghost in a man's body, collapsed uselessly within the uncrossable line, have haunted me for more than forty years. The thing sketched by those lines—left behind within those lines—was me, interrupted, suspended. That creature has grown old along with me, but I like him no better. He has not aged charitably. His bitterness turned to acid, and it can only be said in his favor that he has grown feeble in his rages. Now he tends to babble incoherently in a far corner of my psyche.

But I am not fooled. His disposition mirrors his personality, grim and malevolent. He's arrogant and overbearing and wallows in his insecurities. He is aloof, especially in large groups, the sort who hangs back, observing, criticizing, patronizing when he smells pity, spewing vulgarities if the wrong word is said. Nasty fellow, this ghost of Gary past. I know. I lived with him for twenty or thirty years, listening to him whine, and then one day . . .

After one more convulsion in which the wheelchair became a weapon, after one more fist against a mirror, after one more vile regurgitation of obscenities, after the last stick of frustration was consumed in the smoldering embers of stoicism, this self-styled leper became a burnt-out case.

Then, at last, all the hard-earned knowledge flowered into an existential acceptance of the unfathomable, and the whiner drunk on pity began to appreciate the nature of the unchangeable.

The paralyzed man miraculously found the ability to turn the other cheek, "to live each day fully and gracefully."

. . . .

A July night. A university town. Belinda and I have driven a hundred miles to see a performance of the Texas singer-songwriter Robert Earl Keen, a man whose music provides a joyful chorus as we journey through our lives. The doors to the cavernous beer and dance hall are propped open and we are early, nursing drinks at the small table nearest the stage.

The music begins. Waves of sound from massive amplifiers vibrate my wheelchair. The crowd is mixed, old and young, solitary women of a certain age, obviously married couples, and university students in casual dress.

"Corpus Christi Bay," Keen sings.

The crowd presses closer, and couples begin to dance at its edges. I smell the beer. I hear the cheers and the raucous calls for a favorite song. I watch the cigarette smoke rise and hover as tabletop rubble rains on the floor. The crowd waltzes nearer and nearer the stage.

Keen begins "The Road Goes on Forever."

A loud cheer from the happy army flowers into the lyrics of the familiar song, and every soul closes in on the pulpit from which the joyful noise rings out, dancing, jumping to the beat, embracing the rhythm.

I am surrounded by bliss. I see backs, and hips, and backs of heads. I shout out each verse, my voice rising into the cloud of joyful noise. I am washed in the waves of singers, swimming in a sea of silky summer dresses and soft faded blue jeans, T-shirts, and golden arms. The words, the rhythm pull me upward, outward, and I sail away, sail beyond my past, beyond myself.

And the ghost is left ashore.